# Learning
# by Lists

# Learning
# by Lists

**Dr Stuart McPherson** BSc MBChB MRCP
Senior House Officer in Gastroenterology
Glasgow Royal Infirmary

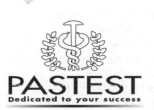

PASTEST
Dedicated to your success

First published 2003

ISBN: 1 901198 30 8

A catalogue record for this book is available from the British Library.

The information contained within this book was obtained by the authors from reliable sources. However, while every effort has been made to ensure its accuracy, no responsibility for loss, damage or injury occasioned to any person acting or refraining from action as a result of information contained herein can be accepted by the publishers or authors.

---

**PasTest Revision Books and Intensive Courses**

PasTest has been established in the field of postgraduate medical education since 1972, providing revision books and intensive study courses for doctors preparing for their professional examinations. Books and courses are available for the following specialties:

**MRCGP, MRCP Part 1 and 2, MRCPCH Part 1 and 2, MRCPsych, MRCS, MRCOG, DRCOG, DCH, FRCA, PLAB.**

For further details contact:

PasTest, Freepost, Knutsford, Cheshire WA16 7BR
**Tel: 01565 752000 Fax: 01565 650264**
**www.pastest.co.uk**  enquiries@pastest.co.uk

---

Cover design by Kingswood Studio, Manchester
Text prepared by Vision Typesetting, Manchester
Printed and bound in Great Britain by Page Bros (Norwich) Ltd

# Contents

# Introduction

This book is a compilation of clinical, diagnostic, investigative and prognostic features of the symptoms and diseases that cover the whole spectrum of general medicine. Reviewed by medical students, this book provides comprehensive lists in the subject areas that commonly appear in their finals. It will be particularly useful for last-minute revision and will also be a useful resource when working on the ward when they come across a clinical problem for which there are a number of possible causes.

Medical student Christina Bell said:

"I genuinely liked the book, and think it will be very popular with students. The idea of learning by lists is officially frowned upon these days in the era of student-directed and problem-based learning, but in reality we need these kind of study aids more than ever before! They help to give us direction and focus our attention on the important and/or commonly asked about areas within medicine.

"I think this kind of book will be most useful for students in their final two years of the medicine course, and especially helpful as a last-minute checklist before clinical examinations, as the lists are concise and to-the-point. They provide answers to the questions which you are asked time and time again as a student on ward rounds and during examinations.

"I have not come across any other resources which cover this area, and I think it definitely fills a gap in the market. These are the kind of lists that we all sit and waste endless hours composing at home, and it is fantastic to have it ready-prepared in such an accessible fashion."

Even though exams do change, lists will remain a vital resource in the candidates' preparation. Although there are several revision books for medical students there have so far been very few that are made up simply of lists. This book aims to fill that gap. Every effort has been made to make the lists as 'user friendly' as possible and they are arranged systematically, the subjects in alphabetical order, with a useful list of abbreviations and a comprehensive index.

Try to memorise as much of each list as possible. You can do this by covering up each heading and reciting the list that follows. Test your colleagues and ask them to test you. If you think that the lists are too long, then break them down into what you think is necessary for your particular needs. Writing your own list will help you to remember more easily.

# List of Abbreviations

| | |
|---|---|
| AAFB | Acid-alcohol-fast bacilli |
| Ab | Antibody |
| ABPA | Allergic bronchopulmonary aspergillosis |
| ACE(I) | Angiotensin-converting enzyme (inhibitor) |
| ACTH | Adrenocorticotrophic hormone |
| AD | Autosomal dominant |
| ADH | Antidiuretic hormone |
| ADP | Adenosine diphosphate |
| AF | Atrial fibrillation |
| AFP | Alphafetoprotein |
| Ag | Antigen |
| ALL | Acute lymphoblastic leukaemia |
| ALP | Alkaline phosphatase |
| ALT | Alanine aminotransferase |
| AML | Acute myeloid leukaemia |
| ANA | Antinuclear antibody |
| APKD | Adult polycystic kidney disease |
| APPT | Activated partial thromboplastin time (with kaolin) |
| AR | Autosomal recessive |
| ARDS | Adult (or acute) respiratory distress syndrome |
| ARF | Acute renal failure |
| AS | Aortic stenosis |
| ASA | Amino salacyclic acid |
| ASD | Atrial septal defect |
| ASOT | Antistreptolysin-O titre |
| AST | Aspartate aminotransferase |
| ATN | Acute tubular necrosis |
| AV | Atrioventricular |
| BCG | Bacillus Calmette–Guérin |
| BTS | British Thoracic Society |

| cANCA | Cytoplasmic-staining anti-neutrophil cytoplasmic antibody |
|---|---|
| CAPRIE | Clopidogrel vs. aspirin in patients at risk of ischaemic events (trial) |
| CAPTURE | Chimeric c7E3 antiplatelet therapy in unstable angina refractory to standard treatment (trial) |
| CCF | Congestive cardiac failure |
| CCK | Cholecystokinin |
| CDC | Centers for Disease Control |
| CEA | Carcinoembryonic antigen |
| CFA | Cryptogenic fibrosing alveolitis |
| CFTR | Cystic fibrosis transmembrane conductance regulator (protein) |
| CHB | Complete heart block |
| CJD | Creutzfeldt–Jakob disease |
| CLL | Chronic lymphocytic leukaemia |
| CML | Chronic myeloid leukaemia |
| CMML | Chronic myelomonocytic leukaemia |
| CMV | Cytomegalovirus |
| CNS | Central nervous system |
| COPD | Chronic obstructive pulmonary disease |
| CPAP | Continuous positive airway pressure |
| CPR | Cardiopulmonary resuscitation |
| CREST | Calcinosis, Raynaud's phenomenon, (o)esophageal dysfunction, sclerodactyly and telangiectasia |
| CRF | Chronic renal failure |
| CRH | Corticotrophin-releasing hormone |
| CRP | C-reactive protein |
| CSF | Cerebrospinal fluid |
| CT | Computed tomography |
| CVA | Cerebrovascular accident |
| CXR | Chest X-ray |
| DEXA | Dual-energy X-ray absorptiometry |
| DIC | Disseminated intravascular coagulation |
| DKA | Diabetic ketoacidosis |
| DMSA | Dimercaptosuccinic acid |
| dsDNA | Double-stranded DNA |
| DTPA | Diethylenetriamine penta-acetic acid |
| DVT | Deep vein thrombosis |
| EBV | Epstein–Barr virus |
| ECG | Electrocardiogram |
| EEG | Electroencephalography |
| ELISA | Enzyme-linked immunosorbent assay |
| EMG | Electromyography |

| | |
|---|---|
| EPIC | Evaluation of 7E3 for the prevention of ischaemic complications (trial) |
| EPILOG | Evaluation in PTCA to improve long-term outcome with abciximab Gp IIb/IIIa blockade |
| EPS | Electrophysiological studies |
| ERCP | Endoscopic retrograde cholangiopancreatography |
| ESM | Ejection systolic murmur |
| ESR | Erthrocyte sedimentation rate |
| ESRF | End-stage renal failure |
| FBC | Full blood counts |
| $FEV_1$ | Forced expiratory volume (in one second) |
| FFP | Fresh frozen plasma |
| FSH | Follicle-stimulating hormone |
| FVC | Forced vital capacity |
| GBM | Glomerular basement membrane |
| GFR | Glomerular filtration rate |
| GGT | Gamma-glutamyltranferase |
| GH | Growth hormone |
| GHRH | Growth hormone-releasing hormone |
| GI | Gatrointestinal |
| GMP | Guanosine monophosphate |
| GN | Glomerulonephritis |
| GORD | Gastro-oesophageal reflux disease |
| GTN | Glyceryl trinitrate |
| HBV | Hepatitis B virus |
| HCG | Human chorionic gonadotrophin |
| HCM | Hypertrophic cardiomyopathy |
| HCV | Hepatitis C virus |
| HHV | Human herpesvirus |
| HIV | Human immunodeficiency virus |
| HLA | Human leucocyte antigen |
| HCM | Hypertrophic obstructive cardiomyopathy |
| HONK | Hyperosmolar non-ketotic state |
| HPV | Human papilloma virus |
| HRT | Hormone replacement therapy |
| HSV | Herpes simplex virus |
| IBS | Irritable bowel syndrome |
| ICP | Intracranial pressure |
| IDA | Iron deficiency anaemia |
| IDL | Intermediate density lipoprotein |
| IFN | Interferon |
| Ig | Immunoglobulin |
| IGF | Insulin-like growth factor |

| | |
|---|---|
| IHD | Ischaemic heart disease |
| INR | International normalised ratio |
| ITP | Idiopathic thrombocytopenia |
| IUGR | Intrauterine growth retardation |
| JVP | Jugular venous pulse |
| LAD | Left axis deviation |
| LBBB | Left bundle branch block |
| LDH | Lactate dehydrogenase |
| LDL | Low density lipoprotein |
| LFT | Liver function test |
| LH | Luteinising hormone |
| LICS | Left intercostal space |
| LPS | Lipopolysaccharide |
| LSE | Left sternal edge |
| LV | Left ventricle |
| LVF | Left ventricular failure |
| LVH | Left ventricular hypertrophy |
| MAC | Membrane attack complex |
| MAG3 | Mercaptoacetyltriglycine (in 99mTc-MAG3) |
| MALT | Mucosa-associated lymphoid tissue |
| MAOI | Monoamine oxidase inhibitor |
| MCGN | Mesangiocapillary glomerulonephritis |
| MCH | Mean corpuscular haemoglobin |
| MCP | Metacarpophalangeal (joints) |
| MCV | Mean corpuscular volume (of red cells) |
| MI | Myocardial infarction |
| MIBG | Metaiodobenzylguanidine |
| MIP | Macrophage inhibitory protein |
| MMR | Measles, mumps and rubella |
| MND | Motor neurone disease |
| MR | Mitral regurgitation |
| MPTP | 1-methyl-4-phenyl-1,2,3,6-tetrahydropyridine |
| MRCP | Magnetic resonance cholangiopancreatography |
| MRI | Magnetic resonance imaging |
| MRSA | Methicillin-resistant *Staphylococcus aureus* |
| MTP | Metatarsophalangeal (joints) |
| MV | Mitral valve |
| MVP | Mitral valve prolapse |
| NADPH | (reduced form of) Nicotinamide-adenine dinucleotide phosphate |
| NHL | Non-Hodgkin's lymphoma |
| NSAID | Non-steroidal anti-inflammatory drug |
| OA | Osteoarthritis |

| | |
|---|---|
| OCP | Oral contraceptive pill |
| PA | Pernicious anaemia |
| PABA | Para-aminobenzoic acid |
| PAN | Polyarteritis nodosa |
| pANCA | Perinuclear-staining anti-neutrophil cytoplasmic antibody |
| PBC | Primary biliary cirrhosis |
| PCOS | Polycystic ovarian syndrome |
| PCP | *Pneumocystis carinii* pneumonia |
| PDA | Patent ductus arteriosus |
| PE | Pulmonary embolus |
| PEA | Pulseless electrical activity |
| PEEP | Positive end-expiratory pressure |
| PEFR | Peak expiratory flow rate |
| PIP | Proximal interphalangeal (joints) |
| PMF | Progressive massive fibrosis |
| PPI | Proton pump inhibitor |
| PS | Pulmonary stenosis |
| PSA | Prostate-specific antigen |
| PSC | Primary sclerosing cholangitis |
| PT | Prothrombin time |
| PTCA | Percutaneous transluminal coronary angioplasty |
| PTH | Parathyroid hormone |
| PTHrP | Parathyroid hormone-related protein |
| PVD | Peripheral vascular disease |
| RA | Rheumatoid arthritis |
| RAD | Right axis deviation |
| RBBB | Right bundle branch block |
| RF | Rheumatoid factor |
| RHF | Right heart failure |
| RICS | Right intercostal space |
| RNP | Ribonucleoprotein |
| RSV | Respiratory syncytial virus |
| RTA | Renal tubular acidosis |
| RVF | Right ventricular failure |
| SBE | Subacute bacterial endocarditis |
| Se HCAT | 23-selena H,25-homotaurocholate |
| sens. | Sensitivity |
| SI | Sacroiliac |
| SIADH | Syndrome of inappropriate ADH secretion |
| SLE | Systemic lupus erythematosus |
| SMA | Smooth muscle antibody |
| spec. | Specificity |
| SSRI | Selective serotonin-reuptake inhibitors |

| | |
|---|---|
| STD | Sexually transmitted disease |
| TG | Triglyceride |
| TIBC | Total iron-binding capacity |
| TLC | Total lung capacity |
| TNF | Tumour necrosis factor |
| TR | Tricuspid regurgitation |
| TRH | Thyrotrophin-releasing hormone |
| TT | Thrombin time |
| TTP | Thrombotic thrombocytopenic purpura |
| TSH | Thyroid-stimulating hormone |
| TV | Tidal volume |
| USS | Ultrasound scan |
| VC | Vital capacity |
| VDRL | Venereal Disease Research Laboratories (test, for syphilis) |
| VIP | Vasoactive intestinal polypeptide |
| VLDL | Very low density lipoprotein |
| VSD | Ventricular septal defect |
| VT | Ventricular tachycardia |
| VZV | Varicella zoster virus |
| WCC | White cell count |
| WPW | Wolff–Parkinson–White syndrome |
| ZN | Ziehl–Neelsen (stain) |

Jo-1, La, Ro and Sm are fractions of nuclear material.

# Cardiology

## Examination

### Pulses

1 Normal
2 Slow-rising pulse – aortic stenosis
3 Collapsing pulse (large amplitude; rapid rise and fall):
   (a) Aortic regurgitation
   (b) Patent ductus arteriosus
   (c) AV shunt
4 Pulsus paradoxus (exaggeration of the normal fall in pulse volume with respiration):
   (a) Cardiac tamponade
   (b) Constrictive pericarditis
   (c) Severe asthma
5 Pulsus bisferiens (double peak):
   (a) Combined aortic stenosis and regurgitation
   (b) Hypertrophic cardiomyopathy
6 Pulsus alternans (alternating large- and small-volume beats):
   (a) Left ventricular failure.

### JVP

#### Waves

1 *a* wave = atrial systole
2 *c* wave = closure of the tricuspid valve
3 *v* wave = atrial filling.

### Abnormalities of the JVP

1  Raised JVP:
   (a)  Right heart failure
   (b)  Fluid overload
   (c)  Superior vena cava obstruction (loss of waves in JVP)
2  Large *a* waves:
   (a)  Pulmonary hypertension
   (b)  Pulmonary stenosis
   (c)  Tricuspid stenosis
3  Absent *a* waves – AF
4  Large *v* waves – tricuspid regurgitation
5  Cannon waves:
   (a)  Complete heart block
   (b)  Extrasystoles
   (c)  Atrial flutter.

## Apex beat (most inferior and lateral cardiac pulsation)

1  Normal:
   (a)  Mid-clavicular line, 5th LICS
2  Displaced laterally:
   (a)  Dilatation of left ventricle (MR, AR, aneurysm) – thrusting
   (b)  Mediastinal shift (pneumothorax etc.)
3  Hypertrophic (heaving) – hypertension
   (a)  AS
   (b)  Coarctation of the aorta
4  Tapping – MS.

## Heart sounds

### First heart sound

Closure of mitral and tricuspid valves.
1  Loud:
   (a)  Mobile mitral stenosis
   (b)  Short PR interval, e.g. WPW syndrome
2  Soft:
   (a)  Immobile mitral stenosis
   (b)  MR
   (c)  Prolonged PR interval.

### Second heart sound

Closure of aortic and then pulmonary valves.
1 Loud:
    (a)  Systemic hypertension (loud A2)
    (b)  Pulmonary hypertension (loud P2)
2 Splitting:
    (a)  Inspiration (physiological)
    (b)  RBBB
    (c)  LBBB (reversed splitting)
    (d)  ASD (fixed splitting; does not vary with respiration).

### Third heart sound

Best heard at left sternal edge or apex.
1 Physiological – due to passive ventricular filling on opening of the AV valves:
    (a)  Young people (<40 years)
    (b)  Hyperdynamic states (e.g. thyrotoxicosis, pregnancy)
2 Pathological – due to rapid ventricular filling:
    (a)  LVF
    (b)  Cardiomyopathy
    (c)  MR
    (d)  VSD
    (e)  Constrictive pericarditis.

### Fourth heart sound

Always pathological. Due to the increased atrial contraction that has to fill a stiff left ventricle. Does not occur in atrial fibrillation.
1 LVH
2 Following MI
3 Amyloid heart disease
4 HCM.

### Murmurs

### Systolic murmurs

1 Mid-systolic murmurs:
    (a)  Innocent flow murmur – soft, short murmur at LSE

  (b) Aortic stenosis or sclerosis – aortic area (2nd RICS), radiating to the neck

  (c) Pulmonary stenosis

  (d) Coarctation of the aorta – coarse murmur maximal over apex of left lung (anterior and posterior)

  (e) Hypertrophic cardiomyopathy – accentuated by the Valsalva manoeuvre

2 Pan-systolic murmurs:

  (a) Mitral regurgitation – apex, radiating to the axilla

  (b) Tricuspid regurgitation (LSE)

  (c) Ventricular septal defect – harsh at LSE

3 Late systolic murmurs:

  (a) Mitral valve prolapse (apex)

  (b) Hypertrophic cardiomyopathy.

## Diastolic murmurs

1 Early diastolic murmurs:

  (a) Aortic regurgitation – maximal 3rd LICS in expiration

  (b) Pulmonary regurgitation

  (c) Graham Steell murmur – pulmonary regurgitation secondary to pulmonary hypertension and mitral stenosis

2 Mid-diastolic murmurs:

  (a) Mitral stenosis – rumbling, mid-late diastole at apex

  (b) Austin Flint murmur (LSE) – aortic regurgitant jet impairing diastolic flow through mitral valve

  (c) Tricuspid stenosis.

## Continuous murmurs

Maximal in systole but persistent into diastole.

1 Parent ductus arteriosus – machinery-like quality at 2nd LICS, mid-clavicular line

2 Venous hum – positional

3 AV shunts/fistulae (in lungs or coronary arteries)

4 Mixed aortic valve disease.

# ECG abnormalities

### Left bundle branch block

Almost always pathological. Wide QRS; M pattern in $V_5$.
1 Ischaemic heart disease
2 LVH
3 Aortic valve disease
4 Cardiomyopathy
5 Myocarditis.

### Right bundle branch block

RSR wave pattern in $V_1$.
1 Normal variant
2 RVH/RV strain (e.g. pulmonary embolus)
3 IHD
4 Congenital heart disease (e.g. ASD)
5 Myocarditis.

### Causes of RVH

1 Cor pulmonale
2 Pulmonary embolism
3 Mitral valve disease
4 Pulmonary hypertension
5 Pulmonary stenosis
6 Fallot's tetralogy.

### Causes of a low-voltage ECG

1 Hypothyroidism
2 COPD
3 Pericardial effusion
4 Dextrocardia
5 Cardiomyopathy.

### Short PR interval

1 Wolff–Parkinson–White syndrome

2  Lown–Ganong–Levine syndrome
3  P wave followed by a ventricular ectopic.

## Wolff–Parkinson–White syndrome

1  Accessory pathway between atria and ventricles
2  Delta wave on ECG
3  Short PR interval
4  Can cause: AF, SVT, VF.

## Prolonged QT interval

Associated with syncope and sudden death (from VT, especially polymorphic VT).
1  Familial (90%):
   (a)  Romano–Ward syndrome (AD)
   (b)  Jervell and Lange–Nielsen syndrome (AR)
2  IHD
3  Metabolic:
   (a)  Hypocalcaemia
   (b)  Hypokalaemia
   (c)  Hypomagnesaemia
4  Drugs:
   (a)  Erythromycin
   (b)  Amiodarone
   (c)  Terfenadine.

## ST depression

1  Myocardial ischaemia (including posterior MI)
2  Digoxin therapy
3  Hypertension
4  LVH with strain.

## ST elevation

1  Myocardial infarction
2  Pericarditis
3  Hyperkalaemia
4  Coronary artery spasm (variant / Printzmetal's angina)
5  Left ventricular aneurysm.

## T-wave inversion

1 Ischaemia
2 Digoxin therapy
3 LVH
4 Cardiomyopathy
5 PE.

## Pulseless electrical activity (PEA; previously electromechanical dissociation or EMD)

Cardiac arrest situation; cardiac rhythm compatible with an output but without any palpable pulse.
 1 Hypo- or hyperkalaemia (or other electrolyte disturbances)
 2 Hypothermia
 3 Hypovolaemia
 4 Hypoxia
 5 Cardiac tamponade
 6 Tension pneumothorax
 7 Pulmonary embolus
 8 Drug/toxin overdose
 9 Aortic dissection
10 Myocardial infarction.

# Arrhythmias

## Tachyarrhythmias

### Sinus tachycardia

1 Anxiety
2 Fever
3 Pregnancy
4 Shock
5 Anaemia
6 PE
7 Thyrotoxicosis
8 Phaeochromocytoma
9 Drugs, e.g. beta-agonists.

### Atrial fibrillation

1 Cardiac causes:
   (a) MI and IHD
   (b) Valvular heart disease (especially mitral stenosis)
   (c) Congenital heart disease
   (d) Cardiomyopathy (especially dilated)
2 Respiratory causes:
   (a) PE
   (b) Pneumonia
3 Others:
   (a) Hypertension
   (b) Hyperthyroidism
   (c) Alcohol (and other drugs)
   (d) Idiopathic ('lone' AF).

### Broad-complex tachycardia

Rate $> 140$ bpm; QRS $> 0.12$ s.
1 Ventricular tachycardia
2 SVT with bundle branch block.

### Junctional tachycardia (SVT)

1 AV nodal re-entry tachycardia, AVNRT (usually structurally normal hearts)
2 AV re-entry tachycardia, AVRT (e.g. Wolff–Parkinson–White syndrome).

### Ventricular tachycardia

1 Myocardial infarction or chronic IHD
2 Myocarditis
3 Cardiomyopathy
4 Hyper- or hypokalaemia
5 Left ventricular aneurysm
6 Prolonged QT interval.

## Features of tachyarrhythmias

**Table 1**

| Type | Rate (bpm) | P wave | QRS complex |
|------|-----------|--------|-------------|
| Sinus | >100 | Normal | Normal |
| Atrial | 120–220 | Abnormal shape | Normal and regular<br>Can have broad complex if aberrant conduction |
| Atrial flutter | 150 | Flutter waves (300/min)<br>Sawtooth pattern | Regular |
| Atrial fibrillation | >120 | Absent | Irregular and normal<br>Can have broad complex if aberrant conduction |
| AVNRT | 140–220 | None seen | Normal, regular |
| AVRT | 140–220 | Inverted P waves after QRS | Normal, regular |
| VT | 120–250 | Dissociated | Broad-complex, regular |

## Bradyarrhythmias

### Sinus bradycardia

Rate 40–50 bpm.
1 Athleticism
2 Myocardial infarction (especially inferior)
3 Hypothyroidism
4 Hypothermia
5 Sinus node disease
6 Raised ICP
7 Increased vagal tone, e.g. vomiting
8 Drugs, e.g. beta-blockers, digoxin, verapamil.

### Heart block

1 First-degree heart block:
   (a) Prolonged PR interval (>0.20 s)
   (b) Usually benign
2 Second-degree heart block:
   (a) Wenckebach (Mobitz 1):
      (i) Successively increasing PR interval until a P wave is not conducted

       (ii)  Usually benign
- (b) Mobitz 2:
  - (i) Unpredictable failure to conduct P waves
  - (ii) Often progresses to complete block
  - (iii) Usually requires a permanent pacemaker
3 Complete heart block (third-degree AV block):
- (a) 25–50 bpm (ventricular escape rhythm)
- (b) Narrow (more stable) or wide QRS complexes
- (c) Associated with large-volume pulse and systolic flow murmurs
- (d) Requires permanent pacemaker
- (e) Causes:
  - (i) Congenital
  - (ii) Acquired
    - Idiopathic fibrosis
    - IHD
    - Acute inflammation (e.g. myocarditis)
    - Chronic inflammation (e.g. sarcoid)
    - Drugs (e.g. rate-limiting agents).

### Indications for permanent pacemakers

1 Complete heart block
2 Mobitz 2 heart block
3 Sinus node dysfunction
4 Symptomatic sinus bradycardia
5 Bifascicular and trifascicular block accompanied by syncope
6 Hypertrophic cardiomyopathy
7 Post AV nodal ablation for arrythmias.

# Ischaemic heart disease

### Risk factors

1 Modifiable:
- (a) Hypertension
- (b) Diabetes
- (c) Smoking
- (d) Hypercholesterolaemia ($\uparrow$LDL, $\downarrow$TG, $\uparrow$HDL)
- (e) Alcohol excess (moderate intake is protective)
- (f) Sedentary lifestyle
- (g) Obesity

(h)  Drugs (contraceptive pill)
2  Fixed:
   (a)  Family history of premature heart disease
   (b)  Chronic renal failure
   (c)  Male gender
   (d)  Increasing age
   (e)  Ethnicity (Afro-Caribbean – low, Indo-Asians – high)
   (f)  Type A personality.

## Management of MI

### *Acute*

1  Oxygen
2  Aspirin
3  GTN
4  Diamorphine
5  Thrombolysis (PTCA if contraindication to thrombolysis):
   (a)  Indications:
      (i)   ST ↑ > 2 mm in two or more chest leads
      (ii)  ST ↑ > 1 mm in two or more limb leads
      (iii) Posterior infarction
      (iv)  New-onset LBBB
   (b)  Contraindications:
      (i)   Bleeding/trauma:
- Internal bleeding
- Heavy vaginal bleeding
- Prolonged or traumatic CPR
- Recent trauma or surgery

      (ii)  Gastrointestinal:
- Acute pancreatitis
- Severe liver disease
- Oesophageal varices

      (iii) Neurological:
- Cerebral neoplasm
- Recent haemorrhagic stroke

      (iv)  Others:
- Active lung disease with cavitation
- Severe hypertension ( > 200/120 mmHg)
- Suspected aortic dissection
- Previous allergic reaction
- Pregnancy or < 18 wks postnatal

CARDIOLOGY

6  Beta-blocker (not if in heart failure)
7  Insulin sliding scale if glucose > 11 mmol/l
8  Diuretics and nitrates if in heart failure
9  ACEI (not if hypotensive)
10 LMWH (prophylaxis of thromboembolism).

### Long-term

1 Risk factor modification:
   (a)  Stop smoking
   (b)  Weight loss
   (c)  Exercise (cardiac rehabilitation)
   (d)  Good diet and reduce alcohol
   (e)  Good diabetic control
   (f)  Treat hypertension
2 Post-infarct prophylaxis:
   (a)  Aspirin ($\downarrow$ vascular events by 29% post-MI)
   (b)  Beta-blockers (reduce mortality by 25% post-MI)
   (c)  Statins (benefit post-MI if cholesterol elevated or normal)
   (d)  ACEI (full-thickness MI or LVF, $\downarrow$ 2-year mortality by 25–30%).

### Complications of MI

1  Arrhythmias (VT/VF, CHB or other AV block)
2  Heart failure/cardiogenic shock
3  Hypertension
4  Thromboembolic disease (DVT/PE, mural thrombus)
5  Pericarditis or Dressler's syndrome
6  LV aneurysm
7  VSD
8  Mitral regurgitation
9  Papillary muscle rupture
10 Cardiac rupture.

# Heart failure

### Causes of heart failure

1 Cardiac causes:
   (a)  IHD

(b) Arrhythmia
(c) Valvular or congenital heart disease
(d) Myocarditis or pericarditis
(e) Cardiomyopathy
2 Drugs:
  (a) Negative inotropes, e.g. beta-blockers
  (b) Fluid-retaining properties, e.g. steroids, NSAIDs
3 Increased metabolic demand:
  (a) Pregnancy
  (b) Hyperthyroidism
  (c) Anaemia
4 Others:
  (a) PE
  (b) Intercurrent illness
  (c) Inappropriate reduction of therapy.

## New York Heart Association classification of heart failure

*Grade 1* – No breathlessness, no effect on daily life
*Grade 2* – breathless on severe exertion
*Grade 3* – breathless on mild exertion
*Grade 4* – breathless at rest, or minimal exertion

## Clinical features of heart failure

1 Symptoms:
  (a) LVF:
    (i) Breathlessness
    (ii) Cough (dry or pink frothy sputum)
    (iii) Cardiac wheeze
    (iv) Orthopnoea and paroxysmal nocturnal dyspnoea
  (b) RVF:
    (i) Peripheral oedema
    (ii) Ascites
2 Signs:
  (a) Left and right:
    (i) Hypotension
    (ii) Tachycardia
    (iii) Gallop rhythm
    (iv) Displaced apex (dilated heart)

   (b) LVF:
       (i)   Bilateral crepitations (lower zones)
       (ii)  Pleural effusions
   (c) RVF:
       (i)   Peripheral oedema
       (ii)  Raised JVP (may have giant *v* waves if TR)
       (iii) Hepatomegaly
       (iv)  Ascites.

## Chest X-ray changes in LVF

1 Upper lobe diversion
2 Cardiomegaly
3 Alveolar oedema
4 Kerley B lines
5 Pleural effusions.

## Treatments for chronic heart failure

1 Low salt diet
2 Fluid restriction
3 Loop diuretics
4 Thiazide diuretics
5 ACE inhibitors (improve survival)
6 Beta-blockers, e.g. bisoprolol, carvedilol (improve survival)
7 Spironolactone (improves survival)
8 Digoxin
9 Vasodilators (nitrates, hydralazine)
10 Anticoagulation
11 Cardiac transplantation.

# Hypertension

## Causes of systemic hypertension

1 Essential hypertension (90%)
2 Renal disease (4%):
   (a) Renal artery stenosis
   (b) Polycystic kidney disease
   (c) Renal parenchymal disease (e.g. glomerulonephritis)

  (d) Chronic renal failure
3 Endocrine disease:
  (a) Diabetes mellitus
  (b) Phaeochromocytoma
  (c) Conn's syndrome (primary hyperaldosteronism)
  (d) Cushing's syndrome
  (e) Acromegaly
  (f) Congenital adrenal hyperplasia
4 Drugs:
  (a) Steroids (including OCP)
  (b) NSAIDs
  (c) Sympathomimetics
5 Pregnancy (pre-eclampsia)
6 Neurogenic (post-head injury)
7 Coarctation of the aorta.

**Complications of systemic hypertension**

1 Cardiac:
  (a) Left ventricular hypertrophy/failure
  (b) IHD
2 Neurological:
  (a) CVA (haemorrhage or infarct)
  (b) Retinopathy
  (c) Hypertensive encephalopathy (rare)
  (d) Increased frequency of subarachnoid haemorrhage
3 Others:
  (a) Aortic aneurysm
  (b) Renal impairment.

# Valvular heart disease

**Mitral stenosis**

1 Causes:
  (a) Rheumatic fever
  (b) Congenital
  (c) Carcinoid
  (d) SLE

2  Clinical signs:
   (a)  Malar flush
   (b)  AF
   (c)  Tapping undisplaced apex
   (d)  Opening snap (mobile valve)
   (e)  Mid-diastolic murmur
   (f)  Evidence of pulmonary hypertension (TR, RV heave, RHF).

## Mitral regurgitation

1  Causes:
   (a)  'Functional', due to LV impairment
   (b)  Rheumatic fever
   (c)  Mitral valve prolapse
   (d)  IHD (post-MI, papillary muscle ischaemia)
   (e)  Endocarditis/myocarditis/cardiomyopathy
   (f)  Connective tissue disorders
   (g)  Collagen disorders (Marfan's syndrome)
2  Signs:
   (a)  AF
   (b)  Displaced hyperdynamic apex
   (c)  Pan-systolic murmur, radiates to axilla
   (d)  Signs of pulmonary hypertension.

## Aortic stenosis

1  Causes:
   (a)  Congenital aortic stenosis
   (b)  Congenitally bicuspid valve
   (c)  Degenerative calcification
   (d)  Rheumatic fever
2  Signs:
   (a)  Slow-rising pulse (narrow pulse pressure)
   (b)  Heaving undisplaced apex
   (c)  ESM radiates to carotids.

## Aortic regurgitation

1  Causes:
   (a)  Congenital (bicuspid or otherwise abnormal valve)
   (b)  Rheumatic fever
   (c)  Infective endocarditis

(d)  Marfan's syndrome
(e)  Syphilis
(f)  Aortic dissection
(g)  Trauma
(h)  SLE
(i)  Hypertension
2 Signs:
  (a)  Collapsing pulse
  (b)  Hyperdynamic undisplaced apex
  (c)  Early diastolic murmur at LSE
  (d)  Corrigan's sign (prominent carotid pulsation)
  (e)  de Musset's sign (head nodding)
  (f)  Quincke's sign (pulsating nail beds)
  (g)  Pistol-shot femorals.

## Tricuspid regurgitation

1 Causes:
  (a)  RV dilatation (pulmonary hypertension, cor pulmonale)
  (b)  Infective endocarditis (intravenous drug users)
  (c)  Rheumatic fever
  (d)  Right ventricular infarction
2 Signs:
  (a)  Giant *v* waves in JVP
  (b)  RV heave
  (c)  Pulsatile hepatomegaly
  (d)  Pan-systolic murmur at LSE (increases on inspiration)
  (e)  Ascites.

# Infective endocarditis

## Predisposing factors

1 Rheumatic heart disease
2 Degenerative heart disease
3 Mitral valve prolapse
4 Intravenous drug use
5 Prosthetic valves
6 Congenital heart disease (bicuspid aortic valve is most common)
7 Hypertrophic cardiomyopathy.

CARDIOLOGY

## Microbiology

1 Viridans streptococci
2 *Streptococcus bovis*
3 *Staphylococcus aureus* (IVDU)
4 Enterococci
5 Gram-negative organisms.

## Clinical features

1 Fever (90%)
2 Anorexia and weight loss
3 New or changing murmur
4 Splinter haemorrhages
5 Clubbing
6 Splenomegaly
7 Petechiae
8 Osler's nodes
9 Janeway lesions
10 Roth spots
11 Systemic emboli
12 Haematuria.

# Congenital heart disease

## Causes of cyanotic congenital heart disease

Right-to-left shunt:
1 Tetralogy of Fallot
2 Complete transposition of the great vessels

Reversal of a previous left-to-right shunt:
3 Eisenmenger's syndrome.

## Causes of acyanotic congenital heart disease

Left-to-right shunt:
1 Ventricular septal defect
2 Atrial septal defect
3 Patent ductus arteriosus

Without a shunt:
4 Congenital aortic stenosis

5 Coarctation of the aorta.

## Atrial septal defect (10%)

1 Three types:
    (a) Ostium secundum (70%) – defect of fossa ovale
    (b) Ostium primum (15%)
    (c) Sinus venosus (15%)
2 Low risk of endocarditis
3 May develop AF
4 Wide fixed splitting of the second heart sound.

## Ventricular septal defect (25–30%)

1 Leads to left-to-right shunt
2 Maladie de Roger is a small defect with a loud murmur
3 Pan-systolic murmur throughout precordium but loudest at LSE
4 Complications:
    (a) SBE
    (b) Pulmonary hypertension and Eisenmenger's syndrome
    (c) Cardiac failure.

## Patent ductus arteriosus (15%)

1 Persistent ductus arteriosus between aorta and pulmonary artery
2 May be closed with indometacin
3 Collapsing pulse and continuous machinery murmur
4 Complications:
    (a) 'Endocarditis' of the ductus
    (b) Eisenmenger's syndrome.

## Tetralogy of Fallot (10%)

1 Usually presents after 6 months of age
2 Four components:
    (a) Pulmonary stenosis
    (b) Right ventricular hypertrophy
    (c) VSD (right-to-left shunt due to the pulmonary stenosis)
    (d) Overriding of the VSD by the aorta
3 Clinical features:
    (a) Cyanotic attacks (due to pulmonary infundibular spasm) with
        syncope (associated with squatting to reduce them)

(b)  Clubbing.

### Coarctation of the aorta (5%)

1  Congential stenosis of aorta (Most are distal to the origin of the left subclavian artery)
2  Associations:
    (a)  Berry aneurysms
    (b)  Turner's syndrome
    (c)  Bicuspid aortic valve
3  Clinical features:
    (a)  Often asymptomatic
    (b)  Hypertension in the upper part of the body
    (c)  Radiofemoral delay
    (d)  Systolic murmur (infraclavicular or posterior)
    (e)  Collateral artery formation (around scapulae or below the ribs posteriorly)
    (f)  May lead to 'endocarditis'.

### Eisenmenger's syndrome

1  Reversal of left-to-right shunt due to development of pulmonary hypertension
2  Occurs in:
    (a)  VSD
    (b)  ASD
    (c)  PDA
3  Clinical features:
    (a)  Central cyanosis
    (b)  Clubbing
    (c)  Decreasing intensity of murmurs (reduced flow)
    (d)  Pulmonary hypertension.

# Causes of syncope

### Cardiac

1  Sinus node disease
2  Atrioventricular disease
3  Tachycardia

4 Bradycardia
5 Myocardial ischaemia
6 Aortic stenosis
7 Hypertrophic cardiomyopathy
8 Pulmonary embolus
9 Aortic dissection

### Neurogenic

1 Epilepsy
2 Vertebro-basilar ischaemia

### Others

1 Hypoglycaemia
2 Vasovagal syncope
3 Postural hypotension:
    (a) Elderly
    (b) Vasodilator drugs
    (c) Parkinson's disease
    (d) Autonomic neuropathy
4 Micturition and cough syncope.

# Cardiomyopathies

### Dilated cardiomyopathy

Global ventricular dilatation and dysfunction.
1 Hereditary (30%) (X-linked, AD)
2 Alcohol
3 Following myocarditis
4 Viruses (coxsackie)
5 Pregnancy
6 Hypertension and IHD.

### Restrictive cardiomyopathy

Stiff, rigid ventricles lead to impaired diastolic filling.
1 Idiopathic
2 Amyloidosis
3 Endomyocardial fibrosis

4  Sarcoidosis
5  Haemochromatosis

**Hypertrophic cardiomyopathy**

Asymmetric hypertrophy of left or right ventricle, or both; autosomal dominant.
1  Clinical features:
   (a)  Breathlessness
   (b)  Chest pains
   (c)  Collapse/syncope
   (d)  Palpitations (AF, SVT, VT)
   (e)  Sudden death
2  Signs:
   (a)  Jerky pulse
   (b)  Forceful apex
   (c)  Ejection systolic murmur (increased by squatting)

# Pericardial diseases

**Acute pericarditis**

1  Post-MI (Dressler's syndrome):
   (a)  Occurs two weeks to two months post-MI or cardiac surgery
   (b)  Fever, pleurisy and pericarditis
   (c)  Antibodies to heart muscle
   (d)  Treat with NSAIDs
2  Infective:
   (a)  Viral (most common) e.g. coxsackie B virus
   (b)  Bacterial (e.g. staphylococcal)
   (c)  TB
3  Hypothyroidism
4  Severe uraemia
5  Malignancy and radiotherapy
6  Trauma
7  Autoimmune (SLE, RA, rheumatic fever)

# Drugs and the heart

[see Table 2, opposite]

**Table 2**

| Drug | Mode of action | Indications | Side effects |
| --- | --- | --- | --- |
| Aspirin | Cyclo-oxygenase inhibitor ↓ Platelet aggregation | Secondary prevention of MI/CVA/PVD | Bleeding, Peptic ulcer, Rash |
| Clopidogrel | ADP-receptor antagonist ↓ Platelet aggregation | Secondary prevention of MI if aspirin intolerant, Coronary stent insertion | Bleeding, Rash |
| Streptokinase, t-PA | Activates plasmin to degrade fibrin | Thrombolysis of MI | Bleeding, Anaphlaxis (streptokinase) |
| Beta-blockers: Atenolol Bisoprolol | ↓ Sympathetic activity Negatively inotropic Negatively chronotropic | Secondary prevention of MI, Anti-anginal, Antihypertensive, Antiarrythmic (AF, SVT, VT), Heart failure | Fatigue, Bradycardia, Bronchospasm, Heart failure |
| Ca antagonists: Verapamil Nifedipine Amlodipine Diltiazem | Block Ca channels on smooth muscle, Vasodilate, Verapamil slows conduction AV and SA nodes | Anti-anginal, Antihypertensive, Antiarrythmic (AF, SVT) – verapamil | Ankle swelling, ↓ LV function, Hypotension |
| Amiodarone | Prolongs cardiac action potential | Antiarrhythmic (all) | Thyroid ↓↑, Photosensitivity, Alveolitis, Hepatitis |

**Table 2** (cont.)

| Drug | Mode of action | Indications | Side effects |
|---|---|---|---|
| Digoxin | Na/K ATPase inhibitor, Slows AV conduction, +ve inotrope | Slowing AF (will not cardiovert) | Any arrhythmia, Nausea, Gynaecomastia |
| Lidocaine (lignocaine) | Blocks Na channels | Antiarrythmic (VT) | Fits, $\downarrow$ LV function |
| Atropine | Anticholinergic | Bradycardia, Asystole | Dry mouth |
| Nitrates | Relax smooth muscle, Venodilators | Antianginal, Heart failure | Headache, Hypotension |
| Thiazides | $\downarrow$ Na reabsorption in proximal tubule | Diuretic, Antihypertensive | $\downarrow$ Na $\downarrow$ K $\downarrow$ Mg, $\uparrow$ urate |
| Furosemide (Frusemide), Bumetanide | $\downarrow$ Na reabsorption in loop of Henle | Diuretic, Heart failure | Dehydration, $\downarrow$ K, Deafness |
| ACE inhibitors: Ramipril Captopril Lisinopril | Inhibit angiotensin-converting enzyme | Heart failure, Post-full-thickness MI, Hypertension, Proteinuria in diabetics | Renal failure, Hypotension, Cough, Angio-oedema, $\uparrow$ K |
| Spironolactone | Aldosterone antagonist | Diuretic, Heart failure, Ascites | $\uparrow$ K, Gynaecomastia |

# Clinical Pharmacology

## Drug metabolism and pharmacokinetics

**Important liver enzyme inducers** (of cytochrome P450, > 200 inducers known)

**PC BRASS**:
1 **P**henytoin
2 **C**arbamazepine
3 **B**arbiturates
4 **R**ifampicin
5 **A**lcohol (chronic)
6 **S**ulphonylureas
7 **S**moking.

**Important drugs whose metabolism is affected by enzyme inducers** (i.e. those metabolised by cytochrome P450 leads to increased metabolism of the drug)

1 Warfarin (↓ INR)
2 OCP (pregnancy)
3 Corticosteroids (↓ effect)
4 All of the enzyme inducers themselves (↓ effect).

**Important liver enzyme inhibitors** (leads to reduced metabolism of the drug and toxicity)

**O DEVICES**:
1 **O**meprazole
2 **D**isulfiram
3 **E**rythromycin

25

4 **V**alproate
5 **I**soniazid
6 **C**iprofloxacin
7 **E**thanol (acute)
8 **S**ulphonamides.

## Important drugs affected by liver enzyme inhibitors

1 Warfarin (↑ INR)
2 Phenytoin (toxicity)
3 Carbamazepine (toxicity)
4 Theophylline (toxicity)
5 Ciclosporin (toxicity).

## Some other clinically important drug interactions

**Table 3**

| Drug | Drug | Effect |
| --- | --- | --- |
| Azathioprine | Allopurinol | Xanthine oxidase inhibition leads to azathioprine toxicity |
| Alcohol | Metronidazole Chlorpropamide | Flushing, hypotension |
| MAOIs | Tyramine Alpha-agonists Amphetamines | Acute hypertensive crisis ('cheese reaction') |
| ACE inhibitors | K-sparing diuretics NSAIDs | Hyperkalaemia Reduced effect of ACEI |
| Digoxin | Thiazides Loop diuretics Amiodarone Nifedipine Verapamil | Digoxin toxicity by ↓ protein binding/renal excretion |
| Beta-blockers | Verapamil | Hypotension and asystole |
| Lithium | Thiazides | Lithium toxicity (↓ excretion) |
| Adenosine | Dipyridamole | Prolonged half-life of adenosine leading to asystole |
| Statins | Fibrates | Increased incidence of myopathy and rhabdomyolysis |
| Aminoglycosides | Loop diuretics | Increased nephrotoxicity and ototoxicity |

## Drugs exhibiting zero-order kinetics (saturation kinetics)

1 Alcohol
2 Phenytoin
3 Fluoxetine

## Examples of drugs that cause their effect by inhibiting enzymes

**Table 4**

| Drug | Enzyme |
| --- | --- |
| ACE inhibitors | ACE |
| Allopurinol | Xanthine oxidase |
| Zidovudine (AZT) | Reverse transcriptase |
| Disulfiram | Aldehyde dehydrogenase |
| MAOIs | MAO |
| Methotrexate/trimethoprim | Dihydrofolate reductase |
| Neostigmine | Cholinesterases |
| Aspirin/NSAIDs | Cyclo-oxygenase |
| Penicillins | Transpeptidase |
| Vigabatrin | GABA transaminase |

**Drugs for which therapeutic monitoring is useful** (i.e. good correlation between blood concentration and therapeutic effect)

1 Digoxin
2 Lithium
3 Aminoglycosides
4 Vancomycin
5 Phenytoin
6 Theophylline.

## Drugs in the elderly

1 Gastric pH↑ , gastric emptying↓, ↓ blood flow – affects absorption of drugs
2 Absorption from intramuscular injections slower due to ↓ muscle mass and ↓ blood flow to muscles
3 Reduced hepatic extraction and metabolism

4  Half-life of some drugs prolonged (e.g. benzodiazepines)
5  Greater volume of fat leads to increased volume of distribution for lipid-soluble drugs
6  GFR reduced in the elderly leading to accumulation of renally excreted drugs (lithium, digoxin etc.)
7  Changes in homeostatic responses make the elderly more susceptible to side effects of some drugs
8  Polypharmacy leads to more interactions.

## Essential features of G6PD deficiency

1  X-linked dominant
2  Present in 5–10% of black men
3  Predisposes to haemolytic anaemia
4  Heterozygotes demonstrate increased resistance to malaria
5  Drugs causing haemolysis in these patients:
   (a)  Primaquine
   (b)  Sulphonamides
   (c)  Sulfasalazine
   (d)  Dapsone.

# Drugs in pregnancy and breastfeeding

## Physiological changes affecting drug metabolism in pregnancy

1  ↑ GFR
2  ↑ Metabolism by P450 enzymes (induction)
3  ↑ Volume of distribution
4  ↓ Protein binding
5  ↓ Gastric emptying.

## Drugs causing teratogenesis (first trimester)

**Table 5**

| Agent | Effect |
| --- | --- |
| Thalidomide | Limb defects, heart defects |
| Anticonvulsants: | |
|    Carbamazepine | Neural tube defects |
|    Phenytoin | Cleft palate, microcephaly, retardation |
|    Valproate | Neural tube defects |
| Cytotoxics | Hydrocephalus, neural tube defects, cleft palate |
| Alcohol | Fetal alcohol syndrome |
| Warfarin | Retarded growth, limb defects, saddle nose |
| Diethylstilbestrol | Adenocarcinoma of vagina (20 years later) |
| Oestrogens | Testicular atrophy in males |
| Anabolic steroids | Masculinisation in females |
| ACE inhibitors | Oligohydramnios, renal failure |
| Retinoids | Hydrocephalus, neural tube defects |
| Lithium | Heart defects |

## Drugs affecting the fetus during intrauterine life and the neonatal period

**Table 6**

| Drug | Effect |
| --- | --- |
| Antibiotics: | |
|    Tetracyclines | Tooth discoloration |
|    Aminoglycosides | Eighth cranial nerve damage |
|    Sulphonamides | Jaundice, kernicterus, neonatal haemolysis and methaemoglobinaemia |
|    Chloramphenicol | Cardiovascular collapse of the newborn ('grey baby syndrome') |
| Antithyroid drugs: | |
|    Iodides | Neonatal hypothyroidism, goitre |
|    Carbimazole | |
| Anticoagulants: | |
|    Warfarin | Fetal and neonatal haemorrhage |
| Hypoglycaemics: | |
|    Sulphonylureas | Fetal and neonatal hypoglycaemia |
| Cardiovascular drugs: | |
|    Beta-agonists | Fetal tachycardia, delayed labour |

CLINICAL PHARMACOLOGY

**Table 6** (*cont.*)

| Drug | Effect |
|---|---|
| Beta-antagonists | Fetal and neonatal bradycardia, neonatal hypoglycaemia, IUGR |
| CNS drugs: | |
|   Alcohol | CNS depression, withdrawal syndromes |
|   Narcotics | |
|   Benzodiazepines | |
|   Lithium | Neonatal hypothyroidism, goitre |
| Corticosteroids and sex hormones | Fetal and neonatal adrenal suppression, virilisation of female fetus |
| NSAIDs: | |
|   Aspirin | Premature closure of ductus arteriosus, delayed labour, increased blood loss, impaired platelet function |
|   Indometacin | |

# Drug side effects

## Drugs that cause direct nephrotoxicity

1 Glomerular damage (GN):
   (a) Penicillamine
   (b) Gold
   (c) Captopril
2 Change renal vascular dynamics:
   (a) ACEIs
   (b) NSAIDs
   (c) Ciclosporin
3 Tubular damage (ATN):
   (a) Amphotericin
   (b) Aminoglycosides
   (c) Cisplatin
   (d) Lithium
4 Interstitial damage:
   (a) NSAIDs
   (b) Sulphonamides.

## Drugs that cause peripheral neuropathy

1 Amiodarone
2 Isoniazid (pyridoxine prevents)
3 Metronidazole
4 Zidovudine (AZT)
5 Vinka alkaloids.

## Drugs that cause convulsions

1 Penicillins
2 Ciprofloxacin
3 All antiepileptics
4 Lidocaine (lignocaine)
5 Lithium.

## Drugs that cause agranulocytosis/neutropenia

1 Carbimazole
2 Zidovudine
3 Clozapine
4 Cytotoxics
5 Captopril.

## Drugs that cause gum hypertrophy

1 Phenytoin
2 Nifedipine
3 Ciclosporin.

Gum hypertrophy may also occur in scurvy, pregnancy and acute promyelocytic leukaemia.

**Drugs that cause jaundice** – see Gastroenterology

# Poisoning

## Antidotes

[see Table 7, overleaf]

**Table 7**

| Drug | Antidote |
|------|----------|
| Benzodiazepines | Flumazenil |
| Beta-blockers | Atropine |
| | Glucagon (7 mg) |
| | Pacing |
| Calcium antagonists | Anticholinergics |
| | Calcium |
| Digoxin | Digoxin-binding antibody |
| Methanol, ethylene glycol | Ethanol infusion |
| Iron | Desferrioxamine |
| Opiates | Naloxone |
| Paracetamol | N-acetylcysteine |
| | Methionine |
| Warfarin | Vitamin K |
| | Fresh frozen plasma |

## Specific Drugs

### *Paracetamol*

1 Physiology:
  (a) In overdose paracetamol oxidised to
      N-acetyl-p-benzoquinonimine (NAPQI)
  (b) Glutathione required to inactivate this toxic metabolite
  (c) In overdose glutathione levels rapidly deplete
  (d) Toxic liver injury occurs from NAPQI
  (e) 12 g or more is potentially serious
  (f) Patients with pre-existing liver disease, alcoholism, anorexia
      nervosa, or those on enzyme-inducing drugs are at higher risk as
      they have lower glutathione stores
2 Features:
  (a) Most are asymptomatic for 24 hours
  (b) Liver damage not detectable until 18 hours
  (c) Hepatic tenderness and abdominal pain on 2nd day
  (d) Maximal liver damage 72–96 hours (hepatic failure)
  (e) Renal failure (ATN) 25%
3 Important prognostic markers:
  (a) PT > 20 s at 24 hours, significant liver damage
  (b) pH < 7.3 after 24 hours = 15% survival

    (c) Creatinine > 300 $\mu$mol/l = 23% survival

    (d) PT > 180 s = 8% survival

4 Management:

    (a) Gastric lavage up to 4 hours

    (b) Methionine or N-acetylcysteine (6% incidence of rash and bronchospasm)

    (c) Liver transplant.

### Salicylates

1 Features:

    (a) Mild to moderate ( < 700 mg/l):

        (i) Deafness and tinnitus

        (ii) Hyperventilation

        (iii) Respiratory alkalosis and metabolic acidosis

    (b) Severe ( > 700 mg/l):

        (i) Confusion

        (ii) Hypotension

        (iii) Cardiac arrest

    (c) Rare complications:

        (i) Non-cardiogenic pulmonary oedema

        (ii) Cerebral oedema

        (iii) Encephalopathy and coma

        (iv) Renal failure

        (v) Hyperpyrexia

        (vi) Hypoglycaemia

2 Management:

    (a) Gastric lavage

    (b) Activated charcoal

    (c) Urine alkalisation with bicarbonate (not forced alkaline diuresis as this may induce pulmonary oedema)

    (d) Haemodialysis

    (e) Supportive measures.

### Tricyclic antidepressants

1 Features:

    (a) Anticholinergic (dry mouth, drowsiness, sinus tachycardia, urinary retention)

    (b) Coma

    (c) Convulsions
    (d) Respiratory depression and hypoxia
    (e) Prolonged QT interval and arrhythmias (aggravated by acidosis)
    (f) Respiratory and metabolic acidosis
    (g) Skin blisters

2 Management:
    (a) Gastric lavage (useful up to 12 hours due to gastroparesis)
    (b) Activated charcoal
    (c) Arrhythmias treated with bicarbonate (i.e. treat acidosis)
    (d) Treat convulsions with diazepam.

## Lithium

1 Features:
    (a) Tremor
    (b) Ataxia
    (c) Dysarthria
    (d) Nystagmus
    (e) Renal failure
    (f) Convulsions
    (g) Circulatory failure
    (h) Coma
    (i) Death

2 Management:
    (a) Gastric lavage (within 6–8 hours)
    (b) Forced diuresis
    (c) Haemodialysis.

# **Dermatology**

## Nails

### Causes of clubbing

1 Lung:
- (a) Carcinoma of the bronchus
- (b) Chronic suppurative lung disease:
  - (i) Bronchiectasis
  - (ii) Lung abscess
  - (iii) Empyema
  - (iv) Cystic fibrosis
- (c) TB
- (d) Mesothelioma
- (e) Cryptogenic fibrosing alveolitis (CFA)
- (f) Asbestosis
2 Heart:
- (a) Congenital heart disease (cyanotic)
- (b) Bacterial endocarditis
3 Gastrointestinal:
- (a) Crohn's/ulcerative colitis
- (b) Cirrhosis
- (c) Tropical sprue
4 Thyroid: acropachy
5 Familial.

### Causes of nail changes

[see Table 8, overleaf]

**Table 8**

| Nail change | Causes |
| --- | --- |
| Pitting and ridges | Psoriasis |
| Onycholysis | Psoriasis |
| | Onychomycosis |
| | Thyroid disease |
| | Trauma |
| Grooves | Acute illness (Beau's lines) |
| | Psoriasis |
| Leuconychia and white bands | Hypoalbuminaemia |
| | Cirrhosis |
| Yellow nails | Yellow nail syndrome |
| Koilonychia | Iron deficiency anaemia |
| Splinter haemorrhages | Trauma |
| | Bacterial endocarditis |
| | Connective tissue disorders (CTDs) |
| Nail fold telangiectasia | CTDs |

# Hair

**Causes of hirsutism** (excess hair occur in androgening-dependent areas)

1  Polycystic ovarian disease
2  Tumours (adrenal, ovarian)
3  Cushing's syndrome
4  Acromegaly
5  Congenital adrenal hyperplasia
6  Androgen therapy and corticosteroids.

**Causes of hypertrichosis** (excess hair in non-androgenic areas)

1  Hypothyroidism
2  Malnutrition
3  Anorexia nervosa (lanugo hair)
4  Underlying malignancy
5  Drugs:
   (a)  Ciclosporin
   (b)  Minoxidil.

# Pigmentation

## Causes of hyperpigmentation

1 Endocrine:
   (a) Addison's disease
   (b) Cushing's syndrome
   (c) Nelson's syndrome
   (d) Pregnancy
2 Metabolic:
   (a) Renal failure
   (b) Cirrhosis
   (c) Haemochromatosis
3 Nutritional (pellagra)
4 Lymphoma
5 Drugs, e.g. amiodarone.

## Causes of hypopigmentation

1 Localised:
   (a) Vitiligo
   (b) Pityriasis versicolor
   (c) Postinflammatory
   (d) Tuberous sclerosis
   (e) Leprosy
2 Generalised:
   (a) Albinism
   (b) Hypopituitarism
   (c) Phenylketonuria.

# Reaction patterns

## Causes of orogenital ulceration

1 Reiter's syndrome
2 Syphilis
3 Gonococcal infection
4 Inflammatory bowel disease
5 Stevens–Johnson syndrome
6 Behçet's disease.

## Common causes of urticaria and angio-oedema

1 Drugs:
   (a) Penicillins
   (b) ACE inhibitors
   (c) NSAIDs
2 Foods, e.g. azo dyes
3 Arthropod reactions
4 Physical stimuli, e.g. increase in body temperature (cholinergic)
5 Plants
6 Systemic diseases (SLE, vasculitides)
7 Animal saliva
8 Inhalants (grass pollens, house dust)
9 C1 esterase inhibitor deficiency (hereditary angio-oedema).

## Causes of livedo reticularis

1 Idiopathic
2 Physiological
3 Vasculitis
4 Hyperviscosity
5 Thrombocythaemia.

## Causes of pyoderma gangrenosum

1 Idiopathic (50%)
2 Inflammatory bowel disease
3 Rheumatoid arthritis
4 Wegener's granulomatosis
5 Leukaemia.

## Causes of erythema nodosum

1 Systemic diseases:
   (a) Sarcoidosis
   (b) Inflammatory bowel disease
   (c) Leukaemia and lymphoma
2 Infections:
   (a) Streptococcal infection
   (b) TB
   (c) Leprosy
   (d) EBV

3  Drugs:
   (a)  Penicillins
   (b)  OCP
   (c)  Sulphonamides.

**Causes of erythema multiforme** (severe systemic form –
Stevens–Johnson syndrome)

1  Idiopathic (50%)
2  Infections:
   (a)  HSV
   (b)  EBV
   (c)  *Mycoplasma*
   (d)  *Streptococcus*
3  Vasculitis (SLE, PAN)
4  Ulcerative colitis
5  Carcinoma and lymphoma
6  Sarcoidosis
7  Pregnancy
8  Drugs:
   (a)  Penicillins
   (b)  Sulphonamides
   (c)  Co-trimoxazole
   (d)  Salicylates.

# Skin manifestations of systemic disease

## Causes of leg ulceration

1  Diabetes mellitus
2  Vascular:
   (a)  Venous insufficiency
   (b)  Peripheral vascular disease
   (c)  Vasculitis
3  Infections:
   (a)  Bacterial infections
   (b)  TB
   (c)  Leishmaniasis
   (d)  Tropical ulcer
4  Trauma

5  Neuropathy
6  Pressure sores
7  Neoplasia
8  Bullous disorders
9  Haemoglobinopathy, e.g. sickle cell disease
10 Pyoderma gangrenosum.

## Skin changes in diabetes mellitus

1  Cutaneous infections
2  Neuropathic ulcers
3  Necrobiosis lipoidica
4  Acanthosis nigricans
5  Xanthomas and xanthelasma
6  Lipoatrophy (porcine insulins)
7  Lipohypertrophy (highly purified human insulins).

# Cutaneous features of some congenital disorders

**Table 9**

| Syndrome | Skin features | Other manifestations |
| --- | --- | --- |
| Tuberous sclerosis (AD) | Angiofibromas, periungal fibromas, shagreen patches, ash-leaf patches | Epilepsy, mental retardation |
| Neurofibromatosis (AD) | *Café-au-lait* spots, axillary freckling, neurofibromas | Acoustic neuromas, sarcoma, iris Lisch nodules, epilepsy |
| Hereditary haemorrhagic telangiectasia (AD) | Facial and mucosal telangiectasia | Epistaxis, GI bleeding |
| Peutz–Jeghers syndrome (AD) | Perioral hyperpigmentation | Multiple GI polyps, intussusception, GI malignancy |
| Ehlers–Danlos syndrome (AD+AR) (defective collagen) | Skin fragility, tissue paper scars, hyperelasticity | Bruising, hyperextensible joints |
| Sturge–Weber syndrome | Facial port-wine stain | Epilepsy, cortical haemangioma, cortical calcification, glaucoma |

# Erythematous and scaly skin disorders

## Common causes of contact dermatitis (patch testing useful)

1 Nickel (jewellery)
2 Epoxy resin (glue)
3 Hair dyes, cosmetics, perfumes
4 Rubber antioxidants (gloves and shoes)
5 Preservatives
6 Plants (primula, poison ivy)
7 Topical drugs (neomycin, local anaesthetics)
8 Sticking plasters.

## Psoriasis

1 35% have a family history
2 Scaly, erythematous plaques affecting any part of the skin
3 Epidermal cell hyperplasia (turnover time reduced from 28 days to 4 days)
4 Arthropathy seen in 8–10% of patients (see Rheumatology)
5 Multiple variants – chronic plaque, scalp, guttate etc.
6 Nails (pitting, ridging, onycholysis)
7 Treatments:
    (a) Topical, e.g. tar, dithranol, steroids
    (b) Systemic, e.g. PUVA (psoralens and UVA), acitretin, methotrexate.

# Blistering skin disorders

## Pemphigoid

1 Autoimmune disorder of the elderly
2 Lesions are large tense blisters (up to 3 cm)
3 Usually on limbs, trunk and mucous membranes
4 Specific antibody (IgG) to the basement membrane of the epidermis in 70%
5 Treat with high-dose prednisolone
6 Complete remission in one year common.

## Pemphigus

1 Autoimmune blistering condition of the epidermis
2 IgG autoantibodies to intracellular material of the epidermis in 90%
   (cf. pemphigoid – Ab to basement membrane)
3 Very fragile blisters which rupture easily (pemphig**us** lesions b**us**t)
4 Mucous membranes often involved – lesions painful
5 Treat with prednisolone or immunosupressants
6 Disease persists for life
7 Mortality 15–20%.

## Dermatitis herpetiformis

1 Intense pruritic vesicular rash on the buttocks and extensor aspect of
   the elbows and knees
2 Associated with coeliac disease
3 IgA deposited in the basement membrane zone
4 Treated with dapsone
5 Gluten-free diet results in slow improvement in rash (1–2 years)
6 Increased risk of lymphoma (reduced by gluten-free diet).

## Infections of the skin

1 Viral:
   (a)  HPV (warts)
   (b)  HSV (cold sores, genital ulceration)
   (c)  VZV (chickenpox, shingles)
   (d)  Molluscum contagiosum (pox virus)
   (e)  Orf (pox virus)
2 Bacterial:
   (a)  *Streptococcus pyogenes:*
        (i)   Impetigo
        (ii)  Erysipelas
        (iii) Cellulitis
        (iv)  Necrotising fasciitis
        (v)   Scarlet fever
   (b)  *Staphylococcus aureus:*
        (i)   Impetigo
        (ii)  Cellulitis
        (iii) Follicular infections
        (iv)  Staphylococcal scalded skin syndrome

(c) *Mycobacterium* (lupus vulgaris)
3 Fungal:
  (a) Candidiasis
  (b) Dermatophytes:
    (i) Tinea pedis (athletes foot)
    (ii) Tinea cruris (groin)
    (iii) Tinea capitis (scalp)
  (c) *Pityrosporum orbiculare* (pityriasis versicolor).

# Malignant tumours of the skin

1 Squamous cell carcinoma:
  (a) On sun-exposed areas
  (b) Ulcerated nodule
2 Basal cell carcinoma:
  (a) Slow-growing papule with rolled edges; can lead to punched-out 'rodent ulcer'
  (b) Most commonly found on the face
3 Malignant melanoma:
  (a) Pigmented lesions
  (b) Metastasises early
  (c) High mortality
4 Lymphoma and leukaemia of the skin
5 Kaposi's sarcoma:
  (a) Purple plaque lesion
  (b) Most common in HIV patients
  (c) Caused by HHV-8.

## Causes of skin tumours

1 UV light
2 Thermal injury
3 X radiation
4 Hydrocarbons
5 Immunosuppression (renal transplantation)
6 HPV
7 HHV-8 (Kaposi's sarcoma)
8 Genetic predisposition (xeroderma pigmentosum)
9 Long-standing skin disease (chronic leg ulcers).

# ━ Endocrinology

## Thyroid disorders

### Thyroid hormones

TRH   Thyrotrophin-releasing hormone
TSH   Thyroid-stimulating hormone
T4/T3 Thyroxine/tri-iodothyronine

**Table 10**

|  | TRH | TSH | T4/T3 |
| --- | --- | --- | --- |
| Type | Peptide | Peptide | Amine (acts like steroid) |
| From | Hypothalamus | Anterior pituitary (basophils) | Thyroid |
| Acts at/via | Intracellular calcium | Cyclic AMP | Nuclear binding |
| Pregnancy | ↑ | ↑ | ↑ |
| Illness |  | ↓ | ↓ |

### Causes of hyperthyroidism (* common)

1 Graves' disease – thyroid-stimulating autoantibodies*
2 Toxic adenoma*
3 Toxic multinodular goitre*
4 Viral (de Quervain's) thyroiditis
5 Postpartum thyroiditis
6 Thyroxine overdose
7 Amiodarone
8 Pituitary adenoma (TSH-secreting) – very rare.

## Causes of hypothyroidism (* common)

1 Autoimmune*:
  (a)  Antimicrosomal antibodies in 90%
  (b)  Antithyroglobulin antibodies in 60%
2 Dietary iodine deficiency
3 Hypopituitarism
4 Drugs*:
  (a)  Carbimazole
  (b)  Lithium
  (c)  Radioactive iodine
  (d)  Amiodarone.

## Clinical features of thyroid disease

**Table 11**

|  | Hyperthyroidism | Hypothyroidism |
|---|---|---|
| Constitutional features | Weight loss | Weight gain |
|  | Heat intolerance | Cold intolerance |
|  | Anxiety | Lethargy |
|  | Clubbing | Hoarse voice |
| Cardiovascular | Tachycardia | Bradycardia |
|  | AF | Pericardial effusion |
|  | Cardiac failure | Cardiac failure |
| Skin | Hair loss | Hair loss |
|  | Sweating | Dry skin |
|  | Pretibial myxoedema (Graves') | Puffy face |
| Menstrual | Amenorrhoea | Menorrhagia |
| Gastrointestinal | Diarrhoea | Constipation |
| Neurological | Tremor | Slow-relaxing reflexes |
|  | Proximal myopathy | Depression |
|  | Psychosis | Poor memory |
|  |  | Carpal tunnel syndrome |
| Blood | ↑ T3 T4 | ↓ T3 T4 |
|  | ↓ TSH | ↑ TSH |
|  | Microcytic anaemia | Macrocytic anaemia |
| Treatment | Beta-blockers | Thyroxine |
|  | Carbimazole |  |
|  | Radioactive iodine |  |
|  | Surgery |  |

## *Eye signs of hyperthyroidism*

**Table 12**

|  | Graves' | Non-Graves' |
| --- | --- | --- |
| Lid lag | ✓ | ✓ |
| Lid retraction | ✓ | ✓ |
| Periorbital oedema | ✓ | ✗ |
| Proptosis and exophthalmos | ✓ | ✗ |
| Diplopia | ✓ | ✗ |
| Optic nerve compression | ✓ | ✗ |

## Thyroid carcinoma

Hardly ever causes hyperthyroidism; 10% of nodules are malignant.
1 Papillary – commonest, least aggressive
2 Follicular – rarer, moderately aggressive
3 Anaplastic – rarest, most aggressive
4 Medullary – arises from C cells
5 Lymphoma – may occur in Hashimoto's thyroiditis.

## Causes of thyroid enlargement

1 Diffuse:
   (a)  Graves' disease
   (b)  Hashimoto's thyroiditis
   (c)  Simple goitre
   (d)  Iodine deficiency
   (e)  Pregnancy
   (f)  Viral thyroiditis
2 Nodular:
   (a)  Nodular goitre
   (b)  Adenoma
   (c)  Thyroid cyst
   (d)  Carcinoma, lymphoma, metastases.

# Adrenal disorders

CRH    Corticotrophin-releasing hormone
ACTH  Adrenocorticotrophic hormone

**Table 13**

|          | CRH          | ACTH                          | Cortisol                   |
|----------|--------------|-------------------------------|----------------------------|
| Type     | Peptide      | Peptide                       | Steroid                    |
| From     | Hypothalamus | Anterior pituitary (basophils) | Adrenal zona fasciculata  |
| Acts via | cAMP         | cAMP                          | Nuclear binding            |

### Cushing's syndrome/disease

Excess adrenocortical hormone production.

### Causes

1 Pituitary tumour (Cushing's disease) – 75–80%
2 Adrenal tumour – 15%
3 Ectopic ACTH (small cell carcinoma, carcinoid) – 5–10%
4 Ectopic CRH (very unusual)
5 Long-term steroid use.

### Features

1 Examination:
   (a)  Obesity and moon face
   (b)  Buffalo hump
   (c)  Hirsutism
   (d)  Acne
   (e)  Thin skin
   (f)  Bruising
   (g)  Hypertension
   (h)  Proximal myopathy
   (i)   Psychosis
2 Investigation:
   (a)  Hyperglycaemia

(b) Hypokalaemia
(c) Hypernatraemia
(d) Osteoporosis.

## Investigations

1 ↑Random cortisol
2 ↑24-hour urinary free cortisol
3 Plasma ACTH (adrenal ↓, ectopic normal or ↑, pituitary ↑)
4 Imaging of pituitary/adrenals
5 Dexamethasone suppression tests.

*High-dose dexamethasone suppression test*

| Normal | Full suppression |
| Pituitary-dependent Cushing's | Some suppression |
| Ectopic ACTH/adrenal tumour | No suppression |

## Hypoadrenalism

Failure of adrenal cortex to produce normal glucocorticoids and mineralcorticoids.
Treatment – replacement hydrocortisone and fludrocortisone (↑ dose in intercurrent infection).

## Causes

1 Autoimmune – Addison's disease (75%)
2 TB (20%)
3 Metastasis
4 Haemorrhage (Friderichsen–Waterhouse syndrome, secondary to meningococcus)
5 Congenital adrenal hyperplasia
6 Pituitary failure
7 Withdrawal of long-term steroids.

## Features

1 History and examination:
   (a) Weakness
   (b) Pigmentation

   (c)  Weight loss
   (d)  Abdominal pain
   (e)  Hypotension
2 Investigations:
   (a)  Hypoglycaemia
   (b)  Hyponatraemia
   (c)  Hyperkalaemia
   (d)  Hypercalcaemia
   (e)  Normocytic anaemia with lymphocytosis
   (f)  Impaired response to short Synacthen® test.

## Congenital adrenal hyperplasia

90% is due to 21-hyroxylase deficiency; 5% is due to 11-hyroxylase
deficiency.
1  Autosomal recessive
2  High ACTH
3  Low mineralocorticoid and cortisol
4  All precursors driven into androgen production, causing virilisation,
   genital ambiguity etc.

## Phaeochromocytoma

Tumour of the adrenal medulla that secretes large amounts of
catecholamines.
1  10% familial
2  10% bilateral
3  10% malignant (i.e. metastasis)
4  10% outside adrenals.

### Features

1  Persistent or intermittent hypertension
2  Tachycardia and palpitations
3  Postural hypotension
4  Headaches
5  Hyperglycaemia and glycosuria
6  Weight loss
7  Change in bowel habit.

### Investigation

1  Urinary metanephrins – vanillymandelic acid (VMA)

2  CT scan
3  MRI (T$_2$-weighted)
4  MIBG scan.

# Hypothalamic and pituitary disorders

## Pituitary hormones

### Anterior

1  ACTH
2  TSH
3  LH
4  FSH
5  GH
6  Prolactin.

### Posterior

1  ADH
2  Oxytocin.

## Pituitary tumours

Microadenoma < 1cm; macroadenoma > 1cm.
Nearly always benign.
50% of all tumours are non-secreting.
Prolactinoma is the most common secreting tumour.

### Features

1  Hypopituitarism (compression or invasion of normal pituitary tissue)
2  Bitemporal hemianopia (compression of optic chiasm)
3  Local mass effect
4  Excess hormone production, e.g. prolactin, GH.

## Prolactin

Excess causes of galactorrhoea, amenorrhoea and hypogonadism.
Under negative control of hypothalamus by dopamine, i.e. *increased* dopamine results in *decreased* prolactin.

### Causes of raised prolactin

1 Prolactinoma
2 Stress, e.g. epileptic fit
3 Pregnancy
4 Oestrogens (oral contraceptive)
5 Dopamine antagonist drugs (metoclopramide, phenothiazines)
6 Polycystic ovary syndrome.

### Causes of low prolactin

Dopamine and dopamine agonists (bromocriptine).

### Prolactinoma

25% of all pituitary tumours.

### Growth hormone

Under control of growth hormone-releasing hormone (GHRH) from hypothalamus, and somatostatin.
Secreted in pulsatile fashion, mainly at night – levels may be undetectable between.
Acts directly and via stimulation of IGF-1 production in the liver.

### Causes of growth hormone deficiency (also hypopituitarism)

1 Pituitary tumours
2 Parapituitary tumour (craniopharyngioma)
3 Trauma (surgery)
4 Infarction
5 Pituitary infection (abscess, TB).

### Features of growth hormone deficiency

1 Decreased energy and exercise tolerance
2 Decreased bone density
3 Reduced muscle mass
4 Increased body fat
5 Increased lipids
6 Reduced cardiac output.

*Features of acromegaly* *(hypersecretion of growth hormone)*

Usually due to pituitary tumour (rarely ectopic GHRH).
12% of all pituitary tumours secrete GH. Of these, 90% are macroadenomas.
Diagnosis by failure of GH to suppress during an oral glucose tolerance test.

1 Examination:
  (a) Coarse facial appearance
  (b) Large hands/feet/hat size
  (c) Enlarged lower jaw
  (d) Carpal tunnel syndrome
  (e) Hyperhydrosis
  (f) Arthropathy
2 Metabolic:
  (a) Hypertension
  (b) Diabetes mellitus
3 Cardiorespiratory:
  (a) Increased cardiovascular mortality
  (b) Obstructive sleep apnoea
  (c) LVH and cardiomyopathy
4 Others – renal stones.

*Treatment of acromegaly* *(also for other pituitary adenomas)*

1 Pituitary surgery (trans-sphenoidal)
2 Octreotide (somatostatin analogue)
3 Pituitary irradiation
4 Bromocriptine.

# Disorders of the sex hormones

## Precocious puberty

### Gonadotrophin-dependent (true) causes

1 Idiopathic
2 CNS/hypothalamic disease (tumour, trauma, infection).

## *Gonadotrophin-independent causes*

1  Congenital adrenal hyperplasia
2  Excess testosterone
3  Adrenal or ovarian tumour
4  Oestrogen therapy
5  Severe hypothyroidism.

## Delayed puberty

1  Overt/occult systemic disease
2  Anorexia
3  Genetic disorders, e.g. Turner's, Klinefelter's, Noonan's, androgen insensitivity.

## Hypogonadism

**Table 14**

| | Causes | Features |
|---|---|---|
| ♂ | Hypopituitarism<br>Selective gonadal deficiency<br>Hyperprolactinaemia<br>Primary congenital gonadal disease:<br>    Klinefelter's, anorchia<br>Primary acquired gonadal disease:<br>    Torsion, castration, radiotherapy<br>    Renal failure, liver failure<br>Androgen receptor deficiency | Loss of libido<br>Increasing pitch of voice<br>Loss of male pattern of hair<br>Decreased testicular size<br>Loss of erectile and<br>ejaculatory function<br>Failure of spermatogenesis<br>Loss of muscle bulk |
| ♀ | Ovarian failure (total):<br>    Dysgenesis<br>    Steroid biosynthetic defect<br>    Oophorectomy<br>    Radio/chemotherapy<br>Ovarian failure (partial):<br>    Polycystic ovary syndrome<br>    Resistant ovary syndrome<br>Gonadotrophin failure:<br>    Hypothalamo-pituitary disease<br>    Anorexia<br>    Systemic illness<br>    hypothyroidism | Thinning and loss of pubic hair<br>Small atrophic breasts<br>Vaginal dryness and dyspareunia<br>Atrophy of vulva and vagina<br>Osteoporosis<br>Infertility<br>Amenorrhoea |

## Causes of gynaecomastia

### Physiological

1 Neonate
2 Puberty
3 Old age.

### Pathological

1 Chronic liver disease
2 Tumours producing oestrogen (adrenal, testicular)
3 Tumours producing HCG (lung, testis)
4 Congenital adrenal hyperplasia
5 Carcinoma of the breast.

### Drugs

1 Oestrogens
2 Digoxin
3 Spironolactone
4 Cimetidine
5 Cyproterone
6 Gonadotrophins
7 Cannabis.

# Disorders of glucose metabolism

## Insulin

1 Peptide hormone
2 Synthesised as proinsulin
3 Cleaved to form insulin and C-peptide on secretion
4 Short plasma half-life
5 Acts via receptor tyrosine kinases
6 Stimulates hepatic glycogen and fat synthesis
7 Stimulates muscle to synthesise glycogen and protein
8 Stimulates adipose tissue to synthesise triglycerides
9 Stimulates uptake of glucose and amino acids by muscle
10 Stimulates cellular uptake of potassium.

## WHO definition of diabetes mellitus (DM)

All definitions are based on venous plasma values of glucose during an oral glucose tolerance test.

**Table 15**

|  | Plasma glucose (mmol/l) | |
|---|---|---|
|  | Fasting | 2 hours post-glucose load |
| Diabetes mellitus | ⩾7.0 | ⩾11.1 |
| Impaired glucose tolerance | <7.0 | 7.8 to 11.0 |
| Normal | <7.0 | <7.8 |

*OR*

Single fasting glucose ⩾ 7.0 mmol/l and characteristic diabetic symptoms.

*OR*

Fasting glucose of ⩾ 7.0 mmol/l on two separate occasions without characteristic symptoms.

## Aetiology of diabetes

### Type 1

1  10% of cases
2  Juvenile onset
3  Insulin-dependent
4  Antibodies to islet cells in pancreas cause autoimmune destruction of insulin-producing cells
5  60–90% have islet cell antibodies at diagnosis
6  50% concordance in identical twins
7  HLA-DR3/4 associated in 95%
8  Commonest in Caucasians.

### Type 2

1  85% of cases
2  Maturity onset
3  Non-insulin dependent
4  Peripheral cell resistance to insulin
5  No associated autoantibodies

6 Identical twins – near 100% concordance
7 70–100% risk if both parents have
8 Commonest in blacks and Asians.

## Secondary diabetes (5%)

1 Due to pancreatic disorders causing insulin deficiency:
  (a) Pancreatitis
  (b) Carcinoma of the pancreas
  (c) Cystic fibrosis
  (d) Haemochromatosis (bronze diabetes)
  (e) Pancreatectomy
2 Due to insulin resistance:
  (a) *Endocrine causes*:
    (i) Cushing's syndrome
    (ii) Thyrotoxicosis
    (iii) Acromegaly
    (iv) Phaeochromocytoma
    (v) Polycystic ovarian syndrome
    (vi) Glucagonoma
  (b) *Drugs*:
    (i) Steroids
    (ii) Thiazides.

## Oral hypoglycaemic agents

### Biguanides (e.g. metformin)

1 Reduce glucose absorption from gut; increase insulin
  sensitivity
2 No weight gain (useful for obese patients)
3 Contraindicated in renal/hepatic failure; may cause
  lactic acidosis.

### Alpha-glucosidase inhibitors (e.g. acarbose)

1 Slow carbohydrate absorption
2 Main side effect is wind.

### Sulphonylureas (e.g. gliclazide)

1 Increase insulin secretion, both basal and stimulated
2 Reduce peripheral resistance to insulin

3  May cause hypoglycaemia (particularly in the elderly)
4  Cause weight gain.

### Thiazolidinediones (e.g. pioglitazone, rosiglitazone)

1  Insulin sensitisers (increase muscle glucose uptake) that reduce peripheral insulin resistance
2  Used in addition to metformin or sulphonylurea
3  Hyperinsulinaemia, hyperglycaemia, hypertriglyceridaemia and Hb $A_{1c}$ levels improved
4  Main adverse effects: hepatotoxicity, weight gain.

## Diabetic emergencies

### Diabetic ketoacidosis (DKA)

1  Usually type 1DM, may be first presentation
2  State of uncontrolled catabolism due to insulin deficiency
3  Usually precipitated by insulin omission or intercurrent illness
4  Vomiting, dehydration, thirst, abdominal pain, hyperventilation, decreased conscious level
5  Ketonuria, hyperglycaemia, metabolic acidosis, hyperkalaemia, may be in renal failure
6  Treat with rehydration, sliding-scale insulin and consider antibiotics and low molecular weight heparin.

### Hyperosmolar non-ketotic state (HONK)

1  Usually type 2 DM
2  Insidious onset
3  May be due to glucose overload or steroid/thiazide treatment in an undiagnosed diabetic
4  Profound dehydration and hyperglycaemia
5  Treatment with rehydration; may have dramatic glucose fall with only a small amount of insulin.

## Hypoglycaemia

### Causes in diabetes

1  Excess insulin/sulphonylurea treatment

2 Inadequate carbohydrate intake.

## Causes unrelated to diabetes

1 Insulinoma
2 Malignancy (due to IGF-2)
3 Adrenal failure
4 Pituitary failure
5 Hepatic failure
6 End-stage renal failure (ESRF)
7 Chronic alcohol abuse
8 Sepsis
9 Post-gastrectomy.

## Complications of diabetes

### Macrovascular

1 Increasing risk of cerebrovascular disease, ischaemic heart disease and myocardial infarction, and peripheral vascular disease
2 Multifactorial: increased age, duration of diabetes, systolic hypertension, hyperlipidaemia and proteinuria
3 Proteinuria strong risk factor for IHD.

### Microvascular

Progress dependent on degree of glycaemic control.

### Retinopathy (see Ophthalmology)

1 Affects 90% at some time
2 Commonest cause of blindness in under-60s
3 Background (early) vs. proliferative (late)
4 After 20 years proliferative retinopathy is found in 60% of type 1 DM patients and 20% of type 2 DM patients.

### Neuropathy

1 Affects 70–90% at some time
2 Huge range of presentations and severity
3 May be due to ischaemia in vasa nervorum.

## Autonomic neuropathy

1 General and gustatory sweating
2 Postural hypotension
3 Gastroparesis
4 Diarrhoea
5 Cardiac arrhythmias.

## Nephropathy

1 Affects 30–40% at some time
2 Commonest cause of death in young diabetics
3 Microalbuminuria = 25–250 mg/day
4 With persistent proteinuria, progression to ESRF is likely in 8–10 years
5 ACE inhibitors slow progression
6 Aggressive control of blood pressure is required.

## Pregnancy and diabetes

Poorly controlled diabetes in the mother is associated with:
1 Fetal macrosomia
2 Intrauterine death
3 Hydramnios
4 Pre-eclampsia
5 Hyaline membrane disease in the newborn
6 Neonatal hypoglycaemia.

DKA carries a 50% mortality rate. Close monitoring important.

## Gestational diabetes

1 Glucose intolerance during pregnancy which remits
   after delivery
2 Usually asymptomatic
3 Treatment with diet, but most will need insulin (oral
   agents may harm the fetus)
4 Likely to recur in subsequent pregnancies
5 Increased incidence of type 2 DM later.

# ▪Gastroenterology

## The mouth

### Causes of mouth ulcers

#### *Local causes*

1 Aphthous ulcers
2 Herpes simplex virus (HSV 1)
3 Coxsackie A virus (hand foot and mouth disease)
4 Trauma
5 Carcinoma (squamous, adenocarcinoma)
6 Idiopathic.

#### *Systemic diseases*

1 Crohn's disease
2 Coeliac disease
3 Glandular fever
4 Tuberculosis
5 Reiter's syndrome
6 Erythema multiforme and Stevens–Johnson syndrome.

### Causes of white oral plaques

1 Candidiasis
2 Squamous cell carcinoma
3 Leukoplakia
4 Hairy leukoplakia.

### Causes of pigmentation of the oral mucosa

1 Addison's disease
2 Peutz–Jeghers disease
3 Lead poisoning
4 Malignant melanoma

5  Drugs, e.g. minocycline.

## Causes of glossitis

1  Nutritional deficiency:
   (a)  Vitamin B$_{12}$
   (b)  Iron
   (c)  Riboflavin
   (d)  Niacin
2  Syphilis
3  Inhalation burns
4  Ingestion of corrosive materials.

## Tongue cancer

1  Squamous cell carcinoma
2  Risk factors:
   (a)  Smoking
   (b)  Alcohol
   (c)  Betel nuts
   (d)  HIV
3  Leukoplakia is precancerous
4  Presents as non-resolving lump or oral ulcer
5  Metastasises to sudmandibular and upper cervical nodes
6  Treatment by excision.

## Causes of bilateral parotid swelling

1  Infections:
   (a)  Mumps
   (b)  Bacterial parotitis
2  Alcoholism and cirrhosis
3  Sjögren's syndrome
4  Sarcoidosis
5  Parotid tumours and lymphoma
6  Amyloidosis
7  Anorexia nervosa and malabsorption.

# Disorder of the upper gastrointestinal tract

## Causes of upper gastrointestinal bleeding

### Common

1 Duodenal ulcer – 35%
2 Gastric ulcer – 20%
3 Gastric erosions – 18%
4 Mallory–Weiss tear – 10%.

### Uncommon (5% or less)

1 Duodenitis
2 Oesophageal varices
3 Oesophagitis
4 Upper gastrointestinal neoplasia.

### Rare (1% or less)

1 Angiodysplasia
2 Hereditary haemorrhagic telangiectasia.

### Causes of dysphagia

1 Obstructive:
   (a) Oesophageal cancer
   (b) Peptic strictures
   (c) Oesophageal web or ring
   (d) Gastric cancer
   (e) Pharyngeal cancer
   (f) Extrinsic pressure, e.g. lung cancer, retrosternal goitre
2 GORD and oesophagitis
3 Hiatus hernia
4 Disordered motility:
   (a) Achalasia
   (b) Systemic sclerosis
   (c) Stroke
   (d) Neurological degenerative conditions, e.g. MND, Parkinson's
5 Pharyngeal pouch

6 Infective:
   (a) Oesophageal candidiasis
   (b) Herpes simplex oesophagitis.

## Oesophageal cancer

1 Squamous or adenocarcinoma (arises from Barrett's epithelium)
2 Mostly middle third
3 Incidence rising
4 50% have metastases at diagnosis
5 5% 5-year survival
6 Risk factors:
   (a) Smoking
   (b) Alcohol
   (c) Achalasia
   (d) Barrett's oesophagus
7 Symptoms:
   (a) Dysphagia for solids, then liquids
   (b) Weight loss
   (c) Pain and dyspepsia
   (d) Haematemesis and melaena
8 Diagnosis:
   (a) Endoscopy
   (b) Barium swallow
   (c) CT and laparoscopy for staging
9 Treatment:
   (a) Surgery
   (b) Endoscopy and stenting
   (c) Radiotherapy
   (d) Chemotherapy (cisplatin and fluorouracil).

## Barrett's oesophagus

1 Complication of long-term gastro-oesophageal reflux
2 Present in 11% of patients symptomatic of GORD
3 Lower oesophageal squamous mucosa replaced with metaplastic columnar mucosa in response to acid
4 Predisposes to adenocarcinoma (30–40-fold increase)
5 Treatment with long-term protein pump inhibitors (PPIs), but this will not reverse it.

## Gastro-oesophageal reflux disease (GORD) and oesophagitis

1 Very common
2 Symptoms:
    (a) Chest pain – retrosternal discomfort
    (b) Dysphagia
    (c) Nocturnal cough and wheeze
    (d) Belching
3 Complications:
    (a) Oesophagitis/ulcer
    (b) Stricture
    (c) Iron deficiency anaemia
    (d) Barrett's oesophagus
    (e) Pulmonary aspiration
4 Aggravating factors:
    (a) Obesity
    (b) Smoking
    (c) Alcohol
    (d) Coffee
    (e) Large meals, particularly fatty food
    (f) Hiatus hernia
    (g) Pregnancy
    (h) Systemic sclerosis
    (i) Drugs – NSAIDs
5 Investigation:
    (a) Symptoms do not correlate with endoscopic appearance (but essential to exclude Barrett's)
    (b) 24-hour pH monitoring (symptoms correlate with low pH)
6 Treatment:
    (a) Lifestyle changes
    (b) Antacids
    (c) $H_2$ antagonists
    (d) PPIs
    (e) Promotility agents – metoclopamide, domperidone
    (f) Fundoplication (open/laparoscopic).

### *Helicobacter pylori*

1 Spiral, flagellate, Gram negative, microaerophilic bacterium
2 Produces urease

3 Diseases associated:
  (a) Gastritis
  (b) DU (95% *H. pylori* +ve)
  (c) GU (80% *H. pylori* +ve)
  (d) Gastric adenocarcinoma and gastric lymphoma
4 Methods of detection:
  (a) Rapid urease test at endoscopy
  (b) Histology
  (c) Culture (useful for sensitivities to antibiotics)
  (d) Urea breath test
  (e) Serology
5 Eradicate with triple therapy, e.g. omeprazole, metronidazole and clarithromycin.

## Causes of gastritis/peptic ulcer disease

1 *H. pylori*
2 NSAIDs and high-dose steroids
3 Alcohol and smoking
4 Stress
5 Zollinger–Ellison syndrome.

## Risk factors for gastric carcinoma

1 Japanese
2 *H. pylori*
3 Pernicious anaemia
4 Chronic atrophic gastritis
5 Male sex
6 Blood group A
7 Gastric resection (increased bile reflux)
8 Nitrosamines in the diet.

## Causes of vomiting

### *Gastrointestinal irritation*

1 Enteritis
2 Drugs – NSAIDs, alcohol, poisons
3 Gastritis/gastric ulcer.

## Obstruction

1 Stricture – malignant, benign
2 Intussusception
3 Volvulus
4 Hernia
5 Paralytic ileus.

## Intra-abdominal inflammation

1 Hepatitis
2 Pancreatitis
3 Appendicitis
4 Pyelonephritis
5 Cholecystitis.

## Metabolic and endocrine

1 Diabetic ketoacidosis/hypoglycaemia
2 Pregnancy
3 Uraemia
4 Hypoadrenalism.

## Neurological

1 Psychogenic
2 Severe pain
3 Drugs (opioids, chemotherapeutic drugs)
4 Migraine
5 Motion sickness
6 Meningitis
7 Ménière's disease
8 Labyrinthitis
9 Raised ICP (benign, malignant).

# Small bowel disorders

## Causes of malabsorption

### Conditions within the gut lumen

1 Lack of pancreatic enzymes:
  (a) Chronic pancreatitis
  (b) Cystic fibrosis
  (c) Pancreatic carcinoma
2 Lack of bile salts:
  (a) Obstructive jaundice
  (b) Bile salt loss
  (c) Bacterial overgrowth
3 Infective:
  (a) Traveller's diarrhoea
  (b) Parasitic disease (especially *Giardia*/helminths)
  (c) HIV
  (d) Tropical sprue
4 Inadequate mixing and motility disorders:
  (a) Post-gastrectomy
  (b) Thyrotoxicosis
  (c) Diabetes (autonomic neuropathy)
  (d) Systemic sclerosis.

### Conditions in the gut mucosa

1 Coeliac disease
2 Disaccharidase deficiency (lactase, sucrase-isomaltase deficiency)
3 Post-infectious malabsorption
4 Crohn's disease.

### Structural disorders

1 Intestinal/gastric resection
2 Radiation enteritis
3 Mesenteric arterial insufficiency
4 Small intestinal lymphoma or other malignancy.

## Tests for malabsorption

**Table 16**

| Test | Use |
| --- | --- |
| Iron/ferritin | ↓ Proximal small bowel disease |
| Folate | ↓ Proximal small bowel disease |
| | ↑ Bacterial overgrowth |
| B₁₂ | ↓ Pernicious anaemia |
| | ↓ Bacterial overgrowth |
| | ↓ Terminal ileal disease |
| | ↓ Chronic pancreatitis |
| | Shilling test useful to differentiate |
| Faecal fat | Steatorrhoea |
| D-xylose test | ↓ Small bowel disease |
| | Normal in pancreatic disease |
| PABA test/ | ↓ Pancreatic disease |
| pancreolauryl test | |
| Hydrogen breath test | ↑ Bacterial overgrowth |
| Duodenal biopsy | Histological diagnosis, e.g. coeliac |
| Jejunal aspirate | Bacterial overgrowth |
| Barium follows-through/ | Structural defects in the small bowel, e.g. |
| small bowel enema | terminal ileal stricture, diverticulae |

## Causes of infective diarrhoea

### Bloody diarrhoea (enterocolitis)

1 *Campylobacter*
2 *Shigella*
3 *Salmonella*
4 *Clostridium difficile*
5 *Escherichia coli* (enteroinvasive)
6 Amoebiasis (*Entamoeba histolytica*)
7 Shistosomiasis.

### Watery diarrhoea

1 Viral – rotavirus, Norwalk virus and adenovirus
2 *Shigella*
3 *Salmonella*
4 *E. coli* (enterotoxigenic)
5 *Vibrio cholerae* – cholera

6  Giardiasis
7  *Cryptosporidium.*

## Causes of non-infective diarrhoea

### Bowel disease

1  Diverticulosis
2  Irritable bowel syndrome
3  Disaccharidase deficiency
4  Carcinoma of bowel
5  Villous adenoma of rectum
6  Post-vagotomy/gastrectomy
7  Inflammatory bowel disease
8  Small bowel malabsorption (see above)
9  Bowel ischaemia
10  Bile acid malabsorption.

### Other causes

1  Thyrotoxicosis
2  Diabetes (autonomic neuropathy)
3  Laxative abuse
4  HIV
5  Drugs:
    (a)  Antibiotics
    (b)  Magnesium-based antacids.

### Coeliac disease

1  Sensitivity to gluten (gliadin fraction) leads to villous atrophy
2  Gluten present in bran, oats, wheat and rye
3  0.1–0.2% of population (greater in the UK – 1 in 300)
4  Clinical features:
    (a)  Diarrhoea
    (b)  Steatorrhoea (vitamin A, D, E and K deficiencies)
    (c)  Weight loss
    (d)  Growth retardation
    (e)  Oral aphthous ulcers
    (f)  Anaemia (folate, iron)
    (g)  Increased incidence of all gastrointestinal malignancy (especially small bowel lymphoma)
    (h)  Dermatitis herpetiformis

(i) Osteomalacia
5 Diagnosis:
   (a) Duodenal/jejunal biopsy
   (b) Endomysial Ab (95% positive predictive value)
6 Treatment with gluten-free diet – recovery of villous atrophy in three months.

# Inflammatory bowel disease (IBD)

Features of Crohn's disease and ulcerative colitis (UC) – see Table 17, overleaf

# Large bowel disorders

### Causes of lower gastrointestinal bleeding

1 Haemorrhoids
2 Anal fissure
3 Diverticulosis
4 Lower gastrointestinal neoplasia – adenomatous polyps, carcinomas
5 Inflammatory bowel disease
6 Infective enterocolitis (above)
7 Ischaemic colitis
8 Angiodysplasia
9 Iatrogenic (endoscopy).

### Causes of constipation

1 Inadequate dietary fibre
2 Functional constipation (IBS)
3 Pregnancy
4 Neoplasm
5 Diverticular disease
6 Immobility
7 Dehydration
8 Crohn's disease
9 Hypothyroidism
10 Hypercalcaemia
11 Pelvic mass
12 Parkinson's disease
13 Hirschsprung's disease
14 Drugs e.g. Opiates.

**Table 17**

| Crohn's disease | Ulcerative colitis |
| --- | --- |
| Affects any part of the gastrointestinal tract from mouth to anus | Always involves rectum and extends confluently into the colon |
| Commonly terminal ileum, colon, anorectum | Terminal ileum may be affected by 'backwash ileitis' |
| 'Skip lesions' of normal mucosa between affected areas | Remainder unaffected |

**Pathology**

| | |
| --- | --- |
| Transmural inflammation | Mucosa and submucosa only involved |
| Non-caseating granuloma (65%) | Mucosal ulcers |
| Fissuring ulcers | Inflammatory cell infiltrate |
| Lymphoid aggregates | Crypt abscesses |
| Neutrophil infiltrates | Loss of goblet cells |

**Clinical**

| | |
| --- | --- |
| Abdominal pain prominent and frequent fever | Diarrhoea, often with blood and mucus |
| Diarrhoea ± blood PR | Urgency and tenesmus |
| Weight Loss | Weight loss |
| Anal/perianal/oral lesions | Fever |
| Fistulae | Abdominal pain less prominent |
| Stricturing common, resulting in obstructive symptoms | |
| Anaemia (Fe, $B_{12}$ or folate deficiency) | |

**Associations**

| | |
| --- | --- |
| ↑Incidence in smokers (50–60% are smokers) | ↓Incidence in smokers (70–80% are non-smokers) |
| Erythema nodosum (5–10%) | ↑Incidence of chronic active hepatitis and sclerosing cholangitis |
| Pyoderma gangrenosum (0.5%) | Other systemic manifestations less common than in Crohn's disease |
| Iritis/uveitis (3–10%) | |
| Joint pain/arthritis (6–12%) | |
| Clubbing | |

**Diagnosis**

| | |
| --- | --- |
| Barium studies: | Barium studies: |
|    cobblestoning of mucosa |    pseudopolyps |
|    rose-thorn ulcers |    loss of haustral pattern |
|    skip lesions |    featureless shortened colon |
| Endoscopy and biopsy | Sigmoidoscopy and biopsy may be sufficient |
| Isotope leucocyte scans useful to diagnose active small bowel disease | |

**Table 17** (cont.)

| Crohn's disease | Ulcerative colitis |
|---|---|
| **Complications** | |
| Fistulae: | Fistulae do not develop |
|   entero-enteral | Toxic megacolon (urgent indication for |
|   entero-vesical | colectomy) |
|   entero-vaginal | Increased incidence of carcinoma – |
|   perianal | 20-fold after 20 years of disease |
| Carcinoma – slightly increased | Preventative colectomy of value |
| incidence of colonic malignancy a | Iron deficiency anaemia |
| Osteomalacia | |
| Abscess formation | |

**Treatment**
5-ASA compounds (sulfasalazine, mesalazine) used for treatment and prevention of relapses
Steroids: topical, oral or parenteral for treatment of flare-up
Azathioprine: prevention of relapse
TNF-alpha antagonists (infliximab): used in severe IBD and Crohn's fistulae
Antibiotics: metronidazole effective
Surgery: recurrence occurs in 30–60% of patients after surgery in Crohn's disease. Surgery in UC (panproctocolectomy) may be curative
Nutritional support

## Colorectal cancer

1 Second most common cancer in the UK
2 Adenocarcinoma arising from tubular or villous adenomatous polyps
3 Commonest in rectum (30%) and sigmoid (30%)
4 Risk factors:
  (a) Inflammatory bowel disease (especially UC)
  (b) Familial polyposis coli (AD)
  (c) Hereditary non-polyposis colon cancer (AD)
  (d) Diet low in fibre
  (e) Diet high in fat and red meat
5 Clinical features:
  (a) Weight loss
  (b) Altered bowel habit
  (c) Abdominal mass
  (d) Right sided:

   (i) Iron deficiency anaemia
   (ii) Abdominal pain
  (e) Left sided:
   (i) Blood PR
   (ii) Altered bowel habit
   (iii) Tenesmus
6 Treatment:
  (a) Surgical resection
  (b) Radiotherapy (to debulk tumour before surgery)
  (c) Adjuvant chemotherapy postop. for Duke's B and C (fluorouracil)
  (d) Carcinoembryonic antigen (CEA) can be used to monitor for recurrence.

## Duke's staging of colorectal cancer

**Table 18**

| Stage | Five-year survival |
| --- | --- |
| A – confined to mucosa and submucosa | 80%+ |
| B – extends through muscularis propria | 60–70% |
| C – regional lymph nodes involved | 30–40% |
| D – distant spread | 0% |

# Liver disorders

## Jaundice

### Prehepatic causes

1 Congenital hyperbilirubinaemia, e.g. Gilbert's syndrome
2 Haemolysis (see Haematology).

### Hepatic causes

1 Alcohol
2 Hepatitis viruses:
  (a) A–E viruses (see below)
  (b) Non A–E viruses
  (c) EBV

(d) CMV
(e) HIV
(f) Arboviruses
3 Drugs (see below)
4 Autoimmune:
   (a) Primary biliary cirrhosis
   (b) Autoimmune (lupoid) hepatitis
   (c) Primary sclerosing cholangitis
5 Inherited conditions:
   (a) Wilson's disease
   (b) Haemochromatosis
   (c) Alpha-1-antitrypsin deficiency
6 Neoplastic:
   (a) Hepatocellular carcinoma
   (b) Liver metastases
7 Others:
   (a) Budd–Chiari syndrome
   (b) Cryptogenic
   (c) Obesity/diabetes (non-alcoholic steatohepatitis)
   (d) Pregnancy
   (e) Right heart failure/constrictive pericarditis
   (f) Connective tissue disease (SLE, scleroderma)
   (g) Shistosomiasis (*Schistosoma* japonicum)
   (h) Leptospirosis.

## Posthepatic causes

*Benign*

1 Gallstones in the bile duct
2 Ascending cholangitis
3 Acute and chronic pancreatitis
4 Biliary stricture
5 Sclerosing cholangitis
6 Retroperitoneal fibrosis
7 Helminthic infections.

*Malignant*

1 Pancreatic carcinoma
2 Cholangiocarcinoma

3  Carcinoma of the ampulla of Vater
4  Carcinoma of the duodenum
5  Hilar lymphadenopathy.

## Viral hepatitis

[See Table 19, opposite]

## Interpretation of hepatitis B serology

1  Hep. B surface Ag (HBsAg) – active infection with hepatitis B, acute or chronic.
2  Hep. B e Ag (HBeAg) – acute infection with hepatitis B or chronic carrier state of high infectivity
3  Hep. B e Ab (Anti-HBe) – resolving acute infection with hepatitis B or a chronic carrier state of low infectivity
4  Hep. B core IgM (Anti-HBc-IgM) – acute infection with hepatitis B
5  Hep. B core Ab (total) (Anti-HBc (total)) – natural infection with hepatitis B at some time
6  Hep. B surface Ab (Anti-HBs) – immunity to hepatitis B – vaccine-induced or natural.

[see Table 20, page 78]

## Primary biliary cirrhosis (PBC)

1  Progressive inflammation and destruction of small bile ducts, leading to cirrhosis
2  Probably autoimmune
3  90% of cases are women
4  Associated with other autoimmune conditions
5  Clinical features:
    (a)  Asymptomatic
    (b)  Cholestatic jaundice
    (c)  Pruritis
    (d)  Xanthelasma (hypercholesterolaemia)
    (e)  Hepatosplenomegaly
    (f)  Portal hypertension
    (g)  Osteomalacia/osteoporosis

**Table 19**

| | Spread | Virus | Clinical features | Treatment | Chronicity | Incubation |
|---|---|---|---|---|---|---|
| A | Faecal–oral | RNA | Anorexia Jaundice Nausea Joint pains Fever | Supportive Benign condition Fulminant hepatitis in 0.2% | No | 15–40 days |
| B | Blood, sexual, vertical | DNA | Asymptomatic jaundice Acute fever Arteritis Glomerulonephritis Arthropathy | Supportive <1% fulminant hepatitis Chronic HBV may respond to interferon Lamivudine | 15–20% (at risk of cirrhosis or HCC) | 50–180 days |
| C | Blood, sexual | RNA | Asymptomatic jaundice Malaise | Fulminant hepatitis rare Chronic HCV may respond to interferon and ribavirin | 60–80% (20% risk of cirrhosis and HCC) | 40–55 days |
| D | Blood (dependent on concurrent HBV infection for replication) | Incomplete RNA | Exacerbates HBV infection and increases risk of hepatic failure and cirrhosis | Interferon of limited benefit | Increases incidence of cirrhosis in chronic HBV | |
| E | Faecal–oral | RNA | Acute self-limiting illness In pregnancy mortality (fetal and maternal) of 25% | Supportive | No | 30–50 days |

6 Diagnosis:
   (a) Antimitochondrial antibodies in 95%
   (b) Predominantly raised ALP (cholestatic picture)
   (c) Liver biopsy – destruction of interlobular ducts, small duct
       proliferation, fibrosis and cirrhosis
7 Treatment:
   (a) Symptomatic therapy
   (b) Transplantation
   (c) Ursodeoxycholic acid may reduce time to transplantation.

**Table 20**

|  | HBsAg | HBeAg | Anti-HBe | Anti-HBc-IgM | Anti-HBc (total) | Anti-HBs |
|---|---|---|---|---|---|---|
| Active infection with hepatitis B | + | + | − | + | + | − |
| Chronic carrier of high infectivity | + | + | − | − | + | − |
| Chronic carrier of intermediate infectivity | + | − | − | − | + | − |
| Chronic carrier of low infectivity | + | − | + | − | + | − |
| Infection with hepatitis B sometime in the past | − | − | ± | − | + | − |
| Natural immunity to hepatitis B | − | − | ± | − | + | + |
| Vaccine-induced immunity to hepatitis B | − | − | − | − | − | + |

## Autoimmune (lupoid) hepatitis

1 Female preponderance 4:1
2 Clinical features: can present with an acute hepatitis or with a chronic
  illness – lethargy, fluctuating jaundice, arthralgia and myalgia
3 Diagnosis:
   (a) Raised IgG
   (b) Hepatitic LFTs
   (c) 80% are ANA or SMA positive
   (d) Liver biopsy is required for diagnosis – interface hepatitis
4 Treatment: steroids to induce remission and azathioprine to maintain
  it.

## Hepatocellular carcinoma

1 Rare
2 Predisposing factors:
   (a) HBV
   (b) HCV
   (c) Cirrhosis (any cause)
   (d) Aflatoxin (carcinogen from the mould *aspergillus flavus*)
3 Diagnosis:
   (a) ↑ AFP (80%) > 500 IU/l – high probability
   (b) USS/CT/MRI of the liver
   (c) Liver biopsy (can cause seeding of the tumour).

## Liver abscess

1 Usually occurs with underlying biliary tract pathology
2 Usually multiple
3 Most frequent organisms are:
   (a) *E. coli*
   (b) *Klebsiella*
   (c) *Proteus*
   (d) *Pseudomonas*
   (e) Anaerobes
4 Presents with spiking fevers and right upper quadrant pain
5 Investigations:
   (a) ↑ WCC
   (b) Abnormal LFTs
   (c) Diagnosis on ultrasound or CT
   (d) Aspiration and culture grows an organism in 90%
6 Treatment:
   (a) Antibiotics – broad-spectrum and guided by culture results
   (b) Aspiration
   (c) Occasionally surgery.

## Drugs that cause jaundice

### *Hepatitis*

1 Paracetamol
2 Rifampicin
3 Isoniazid

4  Diclofenac
5  Valproate
6  Halothane.

### *Cholestasis*

1  Chlorpromazine
2  Erythromycin
3  Oestrogens
4  Penicillins
5  Clavulanic acid.

### Causes of cirrhosis

1  Alcohol
2  Chronic hepatitis B and C virus infection
3  Autoimmune:
   (a)  Primary biliary cirrhosis
   (b)  Autoimmune hepatitis
   (c)  Primary sclerosing cholangitis
4  Inherited:
   (a)  Haemochromatosis
   (b)  Wilson's disease
   (c)  Alpha-1-antitrypsin deficiency
5  Intrahepatic biliary obstruction
6  Extrahepatic biliary obstruction
7  Drugs
8  Cardiac failure
9  Budd–Chiari syndrome
10  Obesity/diabetes
11  Cryptogenic.

### Clinical signs of chronic liver disease

1  Jaundice
2  Finger clubbing
3  Liver flap
4  Leuconychia
5  Palmar erythema
6  Spider naevi
7  Bruising

8 Loss of body hair
9 Gynaecomastia
10 Testicular atrophy
11 Ascites
12 Caput medusae
13 Hepatosplenomegaly
14 Encephalopathy
15 Peripheral oedema
16 Fetor hepaticus.

## Clinical signs of chronic liver disease secondary to alcohol

1 Tremor
2 Parotid enlargement
3 Dupuytren's contracture
4 Pseudo-Cushing's
5 Proximal myopathy
6 Peripheral neuropathy
7 Central neurological signs – Wernicke's encephalopathy/Korsakoff's psychosis
8 Cognitive impairment.

### Other effects of alcohol abuse

1 Neuromuscular:
  (a) Epilepsy
  (b) Polyneuropathy
  (c) Myopathy
  (d) Withdrawal
2 Cardiovascular:
  (a) Cardiomyopathy (dilated)
  (b) Beriberi
  (c) Arrhythmias – AF
  (d) Hypertension
3 Metabolic:
  (a) Gout
  (b) Hyperlipidaemia triglycerides
  (c) Hypoglycaemia
  (d) Obesity
4 Respiratory:

    (a)  Chest infections
    (b)  TB
    (c)  Aspiration pneumonia
5  Haematological:
    (a)  Macrocytosis
    (b)  Thrombocytopenia
    (c)  Leucopenia
6  Bone:
    (a)  Osteoporosis
    (b)  Osteomalacia.

## Grading of hepatic encephalopathy

*Grade 1*
Mild confusion
Agitation
Sleep disorder

*Grade 2*
Drowsiness
Lethargy
Asterixis
Dysarthria

*Grade 3*
Somnolent but rousable
Extensor plantars
Increased reflexes

*Grade 4*
Coma

## Causes of ascites

1  Venous hypertension:
    (a)  Cirrhosis
    (b)  Congestive heart failure
    (c)  Constrictive pericarditis
    (d)  Budd–Chiari syndrome
    (e)  Portal vein thrombosis
2  Hypoalbuminaemia:

(a) Nephrotic syndrome
(b) Malnutrition
3 Malignant disease – secondary carcinomatosis
4 Infections – tuberculous peritonitis
5 Miscellaneous:
   (a) Pancreatic disease
   (b) Ovarian disease
   (c) Myxoedema.

## Physiological changes in the liver in pregnancy

1 Hepatic blood flow remains constant despite an increase in cardiac output, so proportion of cardiac output is reduced from 35% to 29%, affecting drug metabolism
2 Size of the liver remains constant
3 ALP rises 3–4-fold due to placental production
4 Other biochemistry remains the same.

# Disorders of the pancreas

## Acute pancreatitis

### Causes

1 Gallstones
2 Alcohol
3 Trauma
4 Post-ERCP/surgery
5 Viral: mumps, coxsackie B, HIV
6 Hyperlipidaemia
7 Hypercalcaemia
8 Autoimmune – PAN
9 Scorpion venom
10 Drugs: azathioprine, steroids
11 Idiopathic.

### Prognosis

Modified Glasgow prognostic score (validated for gallstones and alcohol) – worse prognosis if more than three of these are present:

1  WBC $> 15 \times 10^9$/l
2  Glucose $> 10$ mmol/l
3  LDH $> 600$ U/l
4  AST $> 200$ U/l
5  Urea $> 16$ mmol/l
6  Calcium $< 2$ mmol/l
7  Albumin $< 32$ g/l
8  $Pao_2 < 8$kpa.

## Chronic pancreatitis

1 Causes:
   (a)  Alcohol
   (b)  Cystic fibrosis
   (c)  Duct strictures
   (d)  Hyperlipidaemia
   (e)  Hereditary
   (f)  Idiopathic
2 Clinical features:
   (a)  Chronic severe pain
   (b)  Weight loss
   (c)  Diabetes
   (d)  Malabsorption
3 Investigations:
   (a)  Calcification on AXR
   (b)  ERCP
   (c)  CT
4 Treatment:
   (a)  Pancreatic enzyme supplements
   (b)  Analgesia
   (c)  Stop alcohol
   (d)  Surgery.

# Genetics

## Single gene disorders

### Autosomal dominant

1  Adult polycystic kidney disease
2  Alpha-1-antitrypsin deficiency
3  Familial polyposis coli
4  Gilbert's syndrome
5  Hereditary spherocytosis
6  Huntington's chorea
7  Marfan's syndrome
8  Myotonic dystrophy
9  Neurofibromatosis
10  Noonan's syndrome
11  Osteogenesis imperfecta
12  Tuberous sclerosis
13  von Willebrand's disease.

### Autosomal recessive

1  Albinism
2  Ataxia telangiectasia
3  Congenital adrenal hyperplasia
4  Cystic fibrosis
5  Friedreich's ataxia
6  Haemochromatosis
7  Homocystinuria
8  Phenylketonuria
9  Sickle cell disease
10  Thalassaemias
11  Wilson's disease.

## X-linked recessive

1  Becker's muscular dystrophy
2  Colour blindness
3  Duchenne muscular dystrophy
4  Glucose-6-phosphate dehydrogenase (G6PD) deficiency
5  Haemophilia A (factor VIII)
6  Haemophilia B (factor IX)
7  Lesch–Nyhan syndrome
8  Retinitis pigmentosa.

## X-linked dominant

Vitamin D-resistant rickets.

## Neurofibromatosis

### Type I

1  1 in 2500
2  Over six *café-au-lait* spots
3  Lisch nodules on the iris
4  Peripheral neurofibromas
5  Axillary freckling
6  Chromosome 17 (*NF1* gene).

### Type 2

1  1 in 35,000
2  Bilateral acoustic neuromas
3  Other cranial and spinal tumours
4  Peripheral schwannomas
5  Fewer peripheral neurofibromas
6  Fewer than six *café-au-lait* spots
7  Chromosome 22 (*NF2* gene).

## Tuberous sclerosis

1  Ash-leaf macules
2  Shagreen patches
3  Adenoma sebaceum
4  Subungual fibromas

5 Low IQ
6 Retinal hamartomas
7 Cardiac rhabdomyomas.

### Marfan's syndrome

1 Tall stature (arm span > height)
2 Arachnodactyly
3 Hyperextendable joints
4 Upward lens dislocation
5 High-arched palate
6 Scoliosis
7 Aortic root dilatation (AR, aortic dissection)
8 Mitral valve prolapse.

# Chromosomal abnormalities

### Kleinfelter's syndrome (47, XXY)

1 1 in 600 males
2 Tall stature
3 Hypogonadism (small atrophic testes)
4 Azoospermia (infertility)
5 Low IQ
6 50% normal testosterone level (↑ gonadotrophins).

### Turner's syndrome (45, XO)

1 1 in 2500 females
2 Streak ovaries
3 Short stature
4 Hypogonadism (low oestrogen, ↑ gonadotrophins, infertility)
5 Osteoporosis
6 Webbed neck
7 Widely spaced nipples
8 Renal abnormalities (e.g. horseshoe kidney)
9 Coarctation of the aorta (10–15%)
10 Normal IQ.

### Triple X syndrome (47, XXX)

1  Tall stature
2  Reduced intelligence
3  Mild developmental and behavioural difficulties.

### Down's syndrome (trisomy 21)

1  1 in 700 live births
2  More common as maternal age increases (1 in 25 over 45 years)
3  Brachycephaly
4  Protruding tongue
5  Single palmar crease
6  Clinodactyly (curved fifth finger)
7  Up-slanting palpebral fissures
8  Epicanthic folds prominent
9  Brushfield spots on the iris
10  Moderate mental retardation
11  Increased incidence of:
    (a)  Cardiovascular malformation, e.g. ASD, VSD
    (b)  Haematological abnormalities (ALL, AML)
    (c)  Early-onset Alzheimers
    (d)  GI abnormalities e.g. Hirschsprung's disease
    (e)  Hypothyroidism
    (f)  Cataracts.

### Edward's syndrome (trisomy 18)

1  Characteristic facies
2  Prominent occiput
3  Overlapping fingers
4  Rocker-bottom feet
5  Congenital heart disease
6  Dislocated hips
7  Renal abnormalities
8  Mental retardation.

### Patau's syndrome (trisomy 13)

1  Microcephaly
2  Cleft lip and palate

3 Polydactyly
4 CNS abnormalities
5 Congenital heart disease
6 Rectal abnormality
7 Mental retardation.

# ▬ **Haematology**

## Red cell disorders

### Features of anaemia

1 Pallor
2 Increased cardiac output:
  (a) Angina
  (b) Flow murmurs
  (c) Palpitations
  (d) Cardiac failure
3 Decreased oxygen-carrying capacity:
  (a) Lethargy
  (b) Breathlessness on exertion.

### Classification of anaemia

Anaemia may be due to either decreased production or increased loss of RBCs.
1 Macrocytic – larger erythrocytes
2 Microcytic – smaller erythrocytes
3 Normocytic – normal-sized cells.

[see Table 21, overleaf]

### Causes of microcytosis

1 Iron deficiency anaemia (IDA) – pencil cells,↓ serum iron ↑TIBC and ↓ ferritin
2 Thalassaemia trait – Mediterranean/Asian origin, check for Hb $A_2$ level (raised)
3 Anaemia of chronic disease – underlying disease is usually obvious.

**Table 21**

| Microcytic, hypochromic | Normocytic, normochromic | Macrocytic |
| --- | --- | --- |
| MCV < 80 fl | MCV 80–95 fl | MCV > 95 fl |
| MCH < 27 pg | MCH > 26 pg | |
| Iron deficiency | Many haemolytic | *Megaloblastic:* |
| Thalassaemia | anaemias | Vit $B_{12}$ deficiency |
| Anaemia of chronic | Secondary anaemia | Folate deficiency |
| disease (some cases) | Acute blood loss | |
| Lead poisoning | Mixed deficiencies | *Normoloblastic:* |
| Sideroblastic anaemia | Bone marrow failure, e.g. | Alcohol, |
| | post-chemotherapy, | Liver disease |
| | infiltration by carcinoma | Hypothyroidism |
| | | Myelodysplasia |
| | | Reticulocytosis |
| | | Haemolysis |
| | | Pregnancy |
| | | Drugs |

## Causes of iron deficiency

1 Chronic blood loss:
   (a) Uterine
   (b) Gastrointestinal
   (c) Haematuria (occasionally)
   (d) Self-inflicted blood loss
2 Increased demands:
   (a) Prematurity
   (b) Growth
   (c) Childbearing
3 Malabsorption:
   (a) Gastrectomy
   (b) Coeliac disease
4 Poor diet.

## Thalassaemia

1 Genetic disorders leading to defective haemoglobinisation of the red cell
2 There are four alpha haemoglobin genes and two beta haemoglobin genes
3 Deletion of genes leads to varying degrees of thalassaemia.

**Table 22**

|  | Clinical syndrome |
|---|---|
| *Alpha genes* | |
| 4 | Normal |
| 3 | Silent carrier – usually phenotypically normal |
| 2 | Thalassaemia minor – usually normal Hb with low MCV |
| 1 | Hb H disease – Hb 8–9, g/dl, low MCV, hypersplenism |
| 0 | Hb Bart's – usually die *in utero* |
| *Beta genes* | |
| 2 | Normal |
| 1 | Thalassaemia minor – usually asymptomatic, ↑ Hb A$_2$, low MCV, Hb 11–12 g/dl |
| 0 | Thalassaemia major – severe anaemia, Hb 2–3 g/dl, need repeated transfusions, splenomegaly, bone deformity due to bone marrow expansion, develop iron overload (see haemochromatosis), ↑ Hb A$_2$, reticulocytosis 4–10% |

## Megaloblastic anaemias

### Causes of folate deficiency

1 Dietary (alcoholics)
2 Increased demand:
   (a) Pregnancy
   (b) Haemolytic anaemias
3 Malabsorption:
   (a) Coeliac disease
   (b) Crohn's disease
   (c) Pancreatic insufficiency
4 Drugs:
   (a) Methotrexate
   (b) Phenytoin.

### Causes of B$_{12}$ deficiency

1 Pernicious anaemia
2 Gastrectomy
3 Terminal ileal disease (Crohn's) or resection
4 Bacterial overgrowth

5 *Diphyllobothrium* infection
6 Dietary (rare).

## Pernicious anaemia

Formation of autoantibodies to parietal cells or intrinsic factor leads to malabsorption of $B_{12}$.

*Clinical features*
1 Lethargy
2 Dyspnoea
3 Glossitis
4 Mild jaundice
5 Peripheral neuropathy
6 Subacute combined degeneration of the cord.

*Associations*
1 Familial
2 Blood group A
3 Vitiligo
4 Myxoedema
5 Hashimoto's thyroiditis
6 Thyrotoxicosis
7 Addison's disease
8 Carcinoma of the stomach.

## Causes of aplastic anaemia

1 Idiopathic – probably autoimmune in most cases
2 Drugs – including chloramphenicol, zidovudine, gold
3 Viral infection – hepatitis C, parvovirus $B_{19}$, EBV
4 Chemo/radiotherapy.

## Features of haemolysis

1 Elevated reticulocyte count (>2%)
2 Jaundice – prehepatic. Unconjugated, water-insoluble bilirubin (therefore NOT found in urine but urobilinogen may be)
3 Abnormal red cell morphology – particularly spherocytes.

## Causes of haemolysis

### Genetic

1 Membrane – hereditary spherocytosis or elliptocytosis
2 Haemoglobin – sickling disorders, thalassemia
3 Enzyme defects – G6PD deficiency.

### Acquired

1 Immune:
   (a) Haemolytic disease of the newborn
   (b) Blood transfusion reaction
   (c) Autoimmune (warm or cold antibody mediated)
   (d) Drug-induced
2 Non-immune:
   (a) Trauma (prosthetic valves)
   (b) Microangiopathic haemolysis (DIC)
   (c) Infection (malaria, septicaemia)
   (d) Hypersplenism.

## Sickle cell disease

1 Abnormal beta chains in haemoglobin leads to Hb S production
2 Hb S becomes insoluble and leads to cell sickling in hypoxic conditions
3 Hb AS = sickle cell trait – mild disease
4 Hb SS = sickle cell disease – severe haemolytic anaemias
5 Common in black Africans
6 Reduced susceptibility to *falciparum* malaria
7 Sickle cell crisis precipitated by:
   (a) Hypoxia
   (b) Infection
   (c) Dehydration
   (d) Systemic illness
8 Crisis leads to:
   (a) Microvascular occlusion and infarction of bone and soft tissues and organs
   (b) Severe pain – due to bone marrow infarction
   (c) Hyposplenism (infarcts)
   (d) Osteomyelitis (*Salmonella*)

(e) Leg ulcers
(f) Renal infarction (papillary necrosis)
(g) Retinopathy
(h) Thrombotic stroke
(i) Pulmonary infarction-chest syndrome
(j) Aplastic crisis – usually precipitated by parvovirus B19 infection.

## Causes of autoimmune haemolytic anaemia

1 *Warm* (autoantibody causes haemolysis at body temperature – usually IgG)
(a) Idiopathic
(b) Secondary:
  (i) SLE and other 'autoimmune diseases'
  (ii) CLL
  (iii) Lymphomas
  (iv) Drugs, e.g. methyldopa
2 *Cold* (autoantibody causes haemolysis well below 37 °C – usually IgM):
(a) Idiopathic
(b) Secondary:
  (i) Infections – *Mycoplasma* pneumonia, infectious mononucleosis
  (ii) Lymphoma
  (iii) Paroxysmal cold haemoglobinuria.

## Causes of polycythaemia

1 Primary – polycythaemia ruba vera
2 Secondary (increased erythropoietin):
(a) Altitude
(b) Chronic lung disease
(c) Cyanotic heart disease
(d) Tissue hypoxia
(e) Obstructive sleep apnoea syndrome
(f) Renal tumours (produce erythropoietin).

### Abnormalities of red cell morphology (poikilocytosis)

| | |
|---|---|
| Pencil cells | IDA (with hypochromic microcytes) |
| Target cells | Liver disease |
| | Post-splenectomy |
| | IDA |
| | Thalassaemias |
| Spherocytes | Any cause of haemolysis |
| | Hereditary spherocytosis |
| Elliptocytes | Hereditary elliptocytosis |
| Sickle cells | Sickle cell diseases (with target cells) |
| Helmet cells and fragmented cells | Microangiopathic haemolysis |
| Polychromasia | Young red cells (implies high reticulocyte count) |
| Howell–Jolly bodies | Splenectomy |

# White cell disorders

### Causes of neutrophilia ($>7.5 \times 10^9$/l)

1 Bacterial infections – generalised/localised
2 Metabolic disorders – acidosis, uraemia, poisoning, eclampsia
3 Corticosteroid therapy
4 Inflammation or necrosis (MI, trauma, vasculitis)
5 Malignant neoplasms
6 Myeloproliferative disorders.

### Causes of lymphocytosis ($>3.5 \times 10^9$/l)

1 Acute viral infections – influenza, glandular fever, acute HIV, mumps
2 Chronic lymphocytic leukaemia
3 Thyrotoxicosis
4 Chronic infections – TB, brucellosis, hepatitis, syphilis
5 Other chronic leukaemias and lymphomas
6 Infancy.

### Causes of eosinophilia ($>0.5 \times 10^9$/l)

1 Allergy – asthma, hay fever, drugs
2 Parasites – ascariasis, toxocariasis

3 Skin diseases – eczema, dermatitis herpetiformis
4 Neoplasms – especially Hodgkin's disease
5 Hypereosinophilic syndrome
6 Miscellaneous, e.g. sarcoidosis, polyarteritis nodosa.

## Causes of monocytosis ($>0.8 \times 10^9$/l)

1 Recovery – especially after chemo/radiotherapy
2 Chronic inflammatory disease, e.g. sarcoidosis, Crohn's, RA, SLE
3 Infections – TB, malaria, brucellosis
4 Hodgkin's disease
5 Myelodysplastic syndromes.

## Causes of neutropenia

1 Associated with viral infections
2 Drug reactions, e.g. carbimazole, zidovudine
3 Collagen diseases, e.g. SLE, rheumatoid
4 $B_{12}$ and folate deficiency
5 Myelodysplasia
6 Marrow infiltration
7 After chemotherapy or radiotherapy
8 Hypersplenism.

# Platelet disorders

## Secondary causes of thrombocytosis (platelets $> 500 \times 10^9$/l)

1 Bleeding
2 Infection
3 Infarction
4 Iron deficiency
5 Trauma
6 Thrombosis
7 Splenectomy.

## Causes of thrombocytopenia

1 Decreased production:
   (a) Marrow failure (seen in leukaemias and myelodysplasias)

(b) Megaloblastosis
(c) Drugs
2 Excessive destruction:
   (a) Immune thrombocytopenic purpura (ITP)
   (b) Viruses
   (c) Drugs
   (d) SLE
   (e) Lymphoma
   (f) Hypersplenism
   (g) Haemolytic uraemic syndrome
   (h) DIC
3 Platelet aggregation – heparin causes this in 5%.

# Causes of pancytopenia

1 Aplastic anaemia (including cytotoxic drug therapy)
2 Bone marrow infiltration (e.g. carcinoma, TB, lymphoma)
3 Leukaemia, some myelodysplasias, myeloma
4 Hypersplenism
5 Megaloblastic anaemia
6 Myelofibrosis.

# Haematological malignancies

1 Leukaemias – acute and chronic
2 Lymphomas
3 Myelodysplasias
4 Myeloproliferative disorders.

### Acute lymphoblastic leukaemia (ALL)

1 An acute leukaemia characterised by lymphoblasts in blood and marrow
2 Predominantly affects children
3 Presents with marrow failure (infection, bleeding etc.)
4 70% cure rate with chemotherapy
5 Further classification is by immunological surface markers.

### Acute myeloid leukaemia (AML)

1 Neoplastic proliferation of myeloid blast cells
2 Presents with marrow failure, leukaemic infiltration and systemic symptoms
3 Predominantly affects adults
4 Bone marrow biopsy for diagnosis
5 Auer rods are common
6 Classified by immunological surface markers
7 20–40% cure rate with chemotherapy
8 Bone marrow transplant also used.

### Chronic myeloid leukaemia (CML)

1 Disease of middle age
2 Presents with tiredness, weight loss and sweating
3 Splenomegaly present in 90%
4 Complications associated with hyperleucocytosis may be found
5 High white cell counts (100–500 × $10^9$/l)
6 Philadelphia chromosome (a balanced translocation between chromosomes 9 and 22, seen in 90% of patients with CML).

### Chronic lymphocytic leukaemia (CLL)

1 Most indolent of chronic leukaemias
2 Many discovered as an incidental finding
3 Commonest cause of lymphocytosis in the elderly
4 Progression through lymphocytosis to lymphadenopathy to hepatosplenomegaly and marrow failure occurs, though many patients may skip stages.

### Hodgkin's lymphoma

1 Presents with lymphadenopathy and systemic symptoms (weight loss, night sweats, fever etc.)
2 Characterised by Reed–Sternberg cells
3 Pain may develop at involved nodes on consumption of alcohol
4 Staging:
*Stage 1* = one group of nodes involved
*Stage 2* = two or more groups of nodes on one side of the diaphragm
*Stage 3* = involvement of nodes on either side of the diaphragm

*Stage 4* = extralymphatic involvement
*Stage A* = no systemic symptoms
*Stage B* = systemic symptoms.

## Non-Hodgkin's lymphomas (NHL)

1 Low grade:
   (a) Relatively mature cells
   (b) Without treatment has an indolent course
   (c) Local radiotherapy often effective
   (d) Single-agent chemotherapy usually used for diffuse disease
2 High grade:
   (a) Cells are immature and disease is progressive without treatment
   (b) Six-month course of combination chemotherapy given
3 Lymphoblastic:
   (a) Cells are very immature and have a propensity to involve the CNS
   (b) Treatment as for ALL.

## Myeloma

1 Plasma cell neoplasm; produces diffuse bone marrow infiltration and focal osteolytic deposits
2 Peak age – 70 years
3 Neoplastic plasma cells produce: IgG (55%), IgA (25%), light chain disease (20%)
4 Symptoms include:
   (a) Bone pain (e.g. back, ribs, long bones, shoulder)
   (b) Renal failure – due to light chain deposition
   (c) Anaemia
   (d) Infection
   (e) Neuropathy
   (f) Amyloid
   (g) bleeding
5 Diagnosis:
   (a) Abundant plasma cells in marrow
   (b) Paraprotein in blood or urine (Bence Jones protein)
   (c) Osteolytic bone lesions
   (d) Supported by ↑ ESR, ↑ calcium, anaemia, 'pepper pot' skull
6 Treatment:
   (a) Supportive (bone pain, transfusion, radiotherapy)

   (b)  Chemotherapy ± autologous bone marrow transplant
7  Prognosis – 50% alive at two years.

# Coagulation disorders

1  Prothrombin time (PT) – measures the extrinsic system and the final
   common pathway – increased with warfarin
2  Activated partial thromboplastin time (APTT) – measures intrinsic and
   final common pathways – increased with heparin
3  Thrombin time (TT) – measures the final part of the common pathway.

## Haemophilia A

1  Deficiency of factor VIII
2  Sex-linked recessive disorder
3  Often presents early in life after trauma/surgery, with bleeds into joints
   or muscles
4  Management includes avoiding NSAIDs and i.m. injections. Minor
   bleeds – desmopressin, pressure and elevation. Major bleeds (e.g.
   haemarthrosis) require factor VIII.

## Coagulation cascades

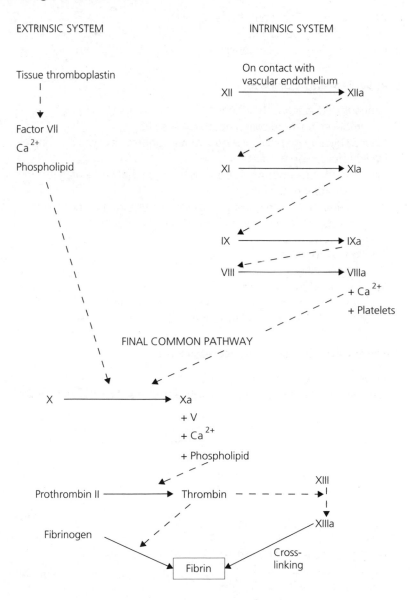

EXTRINSIC SYSTEM

INTRINSIC SYSTEM

Tissue thromboplastin

Factor VII
$Ca^{2+}$
Phospholipid

On contact with
vascular endothelium

XII ⟶ XIIa

XI ⟶ XIa

IX ⟶ IXa

VIII ⟶ VIIIa

+ $Ca^{2+}$

+ Platelets

FINAL COMMON PATHWAY

X ⟶ Xa
+ V
+ $Ca^{2+}$
+ Phospholipid

Prothrombin II ⟶ Thrombin

XIII

XIIIa

Fibrinogen

Fibrin

Cross-
linking

HAEMATOLOGY

## Haemophilia B

1  Also known as 'Christmas disease'
2  Due to factor IX deficiency
3  Clinically similar to haemophilia A.

## von Willebrand's disease

1  Autosomal dominant condition
2  Commonest inherited coagulopathy in the UK
3  Caused by a quantitative or a qualitative abnormality of vWF (von Willebrand factor) production
4  vWF is made on endothelial cells. It is the glue that sticks platelets to damaged subendothelium
5  Disease manifests with bruising, superficial purpura, mennorrhagia, nose bleeds, bleeding from cuts and mucous membranes
6  Diagnosis is made by:
   (a)  Low factor VIII:c
   (b)  Low vWF:Ag
   (c)  Prolonged bleeding time
   (d)  Deficient ristocetin-induced platelet aggregation
7  Treatment is with DDAVP if mild and with vWF concentrate.

## Disseminated intravascular coagulation

1  Caused by release of procoagulant
2  Massive release of coagulation factors and platelets with laying down of fibrin
3  Fibrin immediately removed as the fibrinolytic system put into overdrive, worsening haemmorhagic tendency
4  Laboratory results:
   (a)  Prolongation of APTT, TT, and PT
   (b)  ↑ Fibrin degradation products
   (c)  Thrombocytopenia
   (d)  Microangiopathic blood film
5  Obstetric causes:
   (a)  Retroplacental haemorrhage
   (b)  Retained dead fetus
   (c)  Amniotic fluid embolus
   (d)  Severe pre-eclampsia
6  Other causes:

(a) Crush injury
(b) Septicaemia
(c) Haemolytic transfusion reaction
(d) Malignancy
7 Treatment:
(a) Remove cause
(b) Transfuse with blood, platelets, FFP or cryoprecipitate.

## Risk factors for DVT

1 Increasing age
2 Obesity
3 Immobility
4 Major abdominal surgery
5 Cancer (particularly mucin-producing adenocarcinoma)
6 Trauma to the lower limbs
7 Hormonal:
(a) Pregnancy and the puerperium
(b) Oestrogen/OCP treatment
8 Increased blood viscosity
9 Post-MI or stroke
10 Cigarette smoking
11 Diabetic hypermosmolar state
12 Varicose veins
13 Nephrotic syndrome
14 Inherited:
(a) Presence of factor V Leiden mutation
(b) Protein S or Protein C or antithrombin III deficiency
(c) Family history of thrombosis.

## Thrombophilia

### Congenital causes

1 Deficiencies of:
(a) Antithrombin III
(b) Protein C
(c) Protein S
2 Abnormal prothrombin molecule
3 Dysfibrinogenaemia
4 Fibrinolytic defects

5 Factor V Leiden mutation.

### Acquired causes

1 Polycythaemia and essential thrombocythaemia
2 Lupus anticoagulant/antiphospholipid syndrome.

# The spleen

## Causes of splenomegaly

1 Myeloproliferative disorders:
   (a) Myelofibrosis
   (b) CML
   (c) Polycythaemia rubra vera
   (d) Essential thrombocythaemia
2 Portal hypertension:
   (a) Cirrhosis
   (b) Congestive cardiac failure
3 Chronic haemolytic anaemias:
   (a) Autoimmune haemolytic anaemia
   (b) Cold haemagglutinin disease
   (c) Hereditary spherocytosis
   (d) Haemoglobinopathies
4 Lymphoproliferative disorders:
   (a) Most Lymphomas
   (b) Chronic lymphocytic leukaemia
   (c) Hairy cell leukaemia
5 Infection:
   (a) Bacterial, e.g. typhoid, *Brucella*, TB
   (b) Viral – glandular fever, hepatitis
   (c) Protozoal, e.g. malaria, leishmaniasis
6 Collagen diseases
7 Storage diseases.

# ▬▬ HIV Medicine

## The HIV virus

1 RNA retrovirus
2 Contains enzyme reverse transcriptase
3 Two known types:
   (a) HIV-1 – prevalent worldwide
   (b) HIV-2 – common in West Africa
4 Causes progressive immune dysfunction, characterised by CD4 cell depletion
5 Modes of transmission:
   (a) Sexual intercourse (including oral sex 5%)
   (b) Intravenous drug abuse with shared needles
   (c) Blood and blood products
   (d) Maternal–fetal transmission (also breastfeeding).

## Primary HIV infection (seroconversion illness) – 50%

1 Fever
2 Malaise
3 Diarrhoea
4 Meningoencephalitis
5 Rash
6 Sore throat
7 Lymphadenopathy
8 Arthalgia.

After inoculation seroconversion can take up to six months (the 'window period') and HIV antibody may not be detectable. (Repeat HIV test is therefore required.)

# CDC classification of HIV/AIDS

*Stage 1* – primary seroconversion illness
*Stage 2* – asymptomatic (without treatment – average of ten years before progression to AIDS)
*Stage 3* – persistent generalised lymphadenopathy
*Stage 4* – AIDS

# Indicator diseases for AIDS

1  Recurrent bacterial chest infections
2  Candidiasis (oesophageal, lungs)
3  *Pneumocystis carinii* pneumonia (PCP)
4  Mycobacterial infection (pulmonary TB, extrapulmonary, atypical, Mycobacterium avium-intracellulare complex (MAC))
5  Kaposi's sarcoma
6  CMV disease
7  HSV (ulcers for more than one month or bronchitis, pneumonitis, or oesophagitis)
8  Toxoplasmosis (cerebral)
9  Cryptococcal infection
10  Cryptosporidiosis with diarrhoea for more than one month
11  Isosporiasis with diarrhoea for more than one month
12  Encephalopathy (dementia due to HIV)
13  Progressive multifocal leucoencephalopathy
14  Wasting syndrome (over 10% loss with no other cause identified)
15  Invasive carcinoma of the cervix
16  Recurrent *Salmonella* (non-typhoid) septicaemia,
17  Histoplasmosis – disseminated or extrapulmonary
18  Coccidioidomycosis – disseminated or extrapulmonary
19  Lymphoid interstitial pneumonitis and/or pulmonary lymphoid hyperplasia in a child under 13 years.

# Drug therapies in HIV

### Antiretrovirals

1  Usually started when CD4 $<$ 350 or very high viral load

2 Treatment aims for complete suppression of viral replication
3 Combination therapy with three or four drugs
4 Types:
  (a) Nucleoside reverse transcriptase inhibitors (NRTIs), e.g.
      zidovudine, lamivudine
  (b) Non-nucleoside reverse transcriptases inhibitors (NNRTIs), e.g.
      nevirapine, efavirenz
  (c) Protease inhibitors (PIs), e.g. indinavir, ritonavir.

**Prevention of opportunistic infections**

Co-trimoxazole, pentamidine – PCP prophylaxis (CD4 <200).

# Complications of HIV

**Respiratory complications**

1 Viral infections:
  (a) Adenovirus
  (b) Influenza
  (c) CMV
2 Bacterial infections:
  (a) *Streptococcus pneumoniae*
  (b) *Staphylococcus aureus*
  (c) Tuberculosis:
      (i)   Common presentation
      (ii)  Extrapulmonary disease common
      (iii) Does not tend to have classic CXR
      (iv)  Multi-drug resistance is more common
      (v)   Atypical mycobacterial infections occur,
            e.g. *M. avium-intracellulare* complex
      (vi)  Can occur with any CD4 count
3 *Pneumocystis carinii* pneumonia:
  (d) Common presentation
  (e) Usually occurs when CD4 <200
  (f) Abnormal CXR in 90%
  (g) Hypoxic
  (h) Dry cough, fever, malaise
  (i) Treatment is with high-dose co-trimoxazole

4  Fungal infections:
   (a)  *Candida*
   (b)  *Histoplasmosis*
   (c)  *Cryptococcus*.

## Gastrointestinal complications

### Oropharyngeal/oesophageal disease

99% of patients will develop an oral/oesophageal problem.
1  Candidiasis
2  Oral hairy leukoplakia
3  Aphthous ulcers
4  HSV.

### Diarrhoeal disease

1  Bacteria:
   (a)  *Salmonella*
   (b)  *Campylobacter*
   (c)  *Shigella*
2  Protozoa – *Giardia*, ameobiasis
3  Virus – CMV
4  Opportunistic organisms:
   (a)  Bacteria – MAC
   (b)  Protozoa – *Isospora*, *Cryptosporidia*, *Microsporidia*.

### Pancreatitis

1  CMV
2  Drugs.

### Anorectal conditions

1  HSV
2  Warts (HPV)
3  Syphilis
4  Gonorrhoea
5  *Chlamydia*.

## Neurological complications

1 Can be the first presentation of disease in up to 10%
2 *Mycobacterium tuberculosis* (meningitis, abscess)
3 *Toxoplasma gondii*
4 *Cryptococcus neoformans* (meningitis)
5 CMV (retinitis, peripheral neuropathy)
6 HSV
7 Neurosyphilis
8 AIDS dementia complex
9 Cerebral lymphoma (caused by EBV).

## Ophthalmic complications

1 Uveitis
2 CMV retinitis
3 Toxoplasmosis
4 *Candida* endophthalmitis.

## Neoplastic complications

1 Kaposi's sarcoma (caused by HHV-8)
2 Non-Hodgin's lymphoma
3 Cervical carcinoma
4 Oral squamous carcinoma.

## Dermatological complications

Affect 75% of patients with HIV.
1 Seborrhoeic dermatitis
2 Candidiasis
3 HSV / VZV infections
4 Human papilloma virus
5 Molluscum contagiosum.

# Immunology

## Cells of the immune system

### Polymorphonuclear cells

#### Neutrophils

1  Multilobed nucleus
2  Half life of 6 hours in blood and 1–2 days in the tissues
3  Active in bacterial and fungal infections
4  Attracted to infected tissue by cytokines and bacterial proteins
5  Kill microbes by phagocytosis.

#### Eosinophils

1  Active against multicellular parasites
2  ↑ In allergic patients
3  Can bind IgE
4  Phagocytose Ab–Ag complexes.

#### Mast cells and basophils

1  Basophils circulate in blood
2  Mast cells are active in the tissues
3  Produce histamine, prostaglandins, leukotrienes and proteases
4  Involved in immune response to parasites
5  Immediate hypersensitivity (type I) caused by interaction with Antigen bound to IgE.

#### Mononuclear phagocyte system

1  Monocytes occur in blood
2  Macrophages active in tissue (Kupffer cells, alveolar macrophages and osteoclasts)
3  Functions:

   (a) Cytotoxic (phagocytose opsonised microorganisms – particularly intracellular parasites such as *Mycobacterium tuberculosis*)

   (b) Involved in delayed hypersensitivity reactions (type IV).

## Lymphocytes

### B lymphocytes

1 Mature in bone marrow
2 Form 30% of lymphocytes
3 Express highly specific monoclonal immunoglobulin on their surface
4 When activated there is clonal expansion of the specific B cell, and production of plasma cells (produce antibodies) and memory cells
5 Functions:
   (a) Antibody production
   (b) Antigen presentation
   (c) Produce cytokines to activate T cells.

### T lymphocytes

1 Arise from the thymus gland
2 Form 70% of lymphocyte population
3 Important in intracellular infections, tumour surveillance, and graft rejection
4 T helper cells (66%):
   (a) Have CD4 receptors that interact with MHC class II molecules
   (b) T helper-1 cells:
     (i) Involved in cell-mediated immunity
     (ii) Activate cytotoxic T cells
     (iii) Produce type IV hypersensitivity
   (c) T helper-2 cells:
     (i) Involved in humoral immunity
     (ii) Activate and mature B cells
     (iii) Contribute to type II and III hypersensitivity reactions
5 T cytotoxic/suppressor cells (33%):
   (a) Have CD8 receptors that interacts with MHC class I molecules
   (b) Are important in eliminating cells infected with viruses.

# Immunoglobulins

## IgG

1 Monomer
2 Most abundant in serum
3 Secondary immune response
4 Can cross the placenta.

## IgA

1 Monomer (plasma) or dimer (mucosal surfaces and secretions)
2 Predominantly produced by mucosa-associated lymphoid tissue (MALT)
3 Activates the alternative pathway of complement.

## IgM

1 Pentamer joined by a J chain
2 Primary immune response
3 Very effective agglutinators
4 Opsonises bacteria
5 Includes blood group antibodies.

## IgD

1 Monomer
2 Present on B cells
3 Involved in B-cell activation.

## IgE

1 Involved in type I hypersensitivity reactions (anaphylaxis)
2 Present on mast cells and basophils
3 Rises in response to parasitic infections and in atopic patients.

## Immunoglobulin levels and age

### At birth

IgG: adult levels (active placental transport)
IgA: absent (increased levels suggest acquired *in-utero* infection)

IgM: absent (increased levels suggest acquired *in-utero* infection).
IgG: levels fall at 3–6 months (prone to infection)

### *Adult levels*

IgM: 1 year
IgG: 5–6 years
IgA: puberty

# Complement

1  Postive-feedback enzymic cascade of $>$ 40 proteins
2  Complement mainly made in the liver
3  Functions:
   (a)  Opsonisation and lysis of bacteria
   (b)  Production of proinflammatory mediators
   (c)  Solubilisation of antibody–antigen complexes
4  Classical pathway: initiated by Ab–Ag complexes
5  Alternative pathway activated by:
   (a)  Endotoxin
   (b)  Bacterial cell walls
   (c)  IgA
6  Membrane attack pathway:
   (a)  Final common pathway
   (b)  Generates the more biologically active components such as C5a
      and the membrane attack complex (MAC)
7  Membrane attack complex:
   (a)  Structure that makes holes in cell membranes
   (b)  Causes lysis of cell membranes and cell death.

# Hypersensitivity reactions

### Type I (anaphylactic)

1  Immediate ($<$ 30 minutes)
2  IgE-mediated
3  Specific Ag + IgE + mast cell/basophil = vasoactive mediator release
4  Systemic reaction leads to anaphylaxis

5 Local reactions lead to atopy – asthma, hay fever, eczema, allergic rhinitis.

## Type II (cytotoxic)

1 Mediated by IgG and IgM antibodies
2 Ig + tissue Ag = complement activation, lysis, opsonisation, phagocytosis and inflammation
3 Neutrophils attracted
4 Examples include:
   (a) Transfusion reactions
   (b) Haemolytic disease of the newborn
   (c) Idiopathic thrombocytopenia
   (d) Haemolytic anaemia.

## Type III (immune complex)

1 Circulating antibody that reacts with free antigen, forming immune complexes
2 Ig–Ag deposits lead to complement, mast cell and neutrophil activation
3 Leads to:
   (a) Vasculitis (complexes deposited in vessels)
   (b) Nephritis (complexes deposited in kidneys)
   (c) Extrinsic allergic alveolitis (complexes deposited in lungs)
4 Examples include:
   (a) Arthus reaction
   (b) SLE
   (c) RA
   (d) Glomerulonephritis
   (e) Extrinsic allergic alveolitis.

## Type IV (delayed hypersensitivity)

1 Involves cell-mediated cytotoxicity (CD4 T cells), mediator release and macrophage activation
2 Reaction after more than 12 hours
3 Leads to granuloma formation
4 Examples include:
   (a) TB
   (b) Mantoux test

(c) Graft rejection
(d) Contact dermatitis.

## Major histocompatibility complex (MHC)

1 Genes expressed on short arm of chromosome 6
2 Codes for human leucocyte antigens (HLA)
3 HLA are molecules involved in antigen recognition by T lymphocytes
4 T lymphocytes will only recognise antigen that is presented by an HLA molecule
5 Class I:
    (a) A, B, C
    (b) Signals that the carrier cell is 'infected' and suitable for destruction
    (c) Only interacts with CD8 cytotoxic T cells
6 Class II:
    (a) DP, DQ, DR
    (b) Interacts with CD4 T helper cells to protect against cytotoxic T cells.

# Transplantation

## Types of transplant

1 Autograft – transplant within one individual
2 Syngraft – transplant between genetically identical individuals
3 Allograft – transplant between non-identical individuals
4 Xenograft – transplant between species.

## Rejection

**Table 23**

| Type | Time | Pathophysiology |
|------|------|-----------------|
| Hyperacute | Minutes | Due to preformed antibodies, i.e. ABO mismatch or antibodies to HLA class I molecules from previous transfusion or transplant |
| Acute | < 10 days | Mediated by CD8 cytotoxic T cells |
| Chronic | Years | Unclear. Could be due to immune complex deposition and complement activation |

# Vaccines

## Current immunisation guidelines (Sept 2002)

### At two, three and four months

1 Triple vaccine (diphtheria, tetanus, pertussis)
2 Hib (*Haemophilus influenzae* b)
3 Meningococcal C
4 Polio
5 (BCG in high-risk children).

### At twelve to fifteen months

MMR (measles, mumps and rubella).

### At four to five years

1 Polio booster
2 Diphtheria and tetanus booster
3 MMR booster.

### At ten to fourteen years

BCG (bacillus Calmette–Guérin).

### At fifteen to eighteen years

1 Diphtheria and tetanus booster
2 Polio booster.

### Adulthood

1 Rubella in women seronegative for rubella
2 Tetanus ten-yearly.

# The acute phase response

1 Normocytic anaemia
2 ↑ Immunoglobulins
3 ↑ CRP

4 ↑ Serum amyloid P component (AP)
5 ↑ Ferritin
6 ↑ Fibrinogen leads to ↑ ESR
7 ↑ ALP
8 ↓ Albumin
9 ↑ Platelets
10 ↑ Complement
11 ↑ Caeruloplasmin
12 ↑ Alpha-1-antitrypsin
13 ↑ Angiotensin
14 ↑ Haptoglobin.

# Autoantibodies in autoimmune disease

**Table 24**

| Disease | Antigen |
| --- | --- |
| Hashimoto's thyroiditis | Thyroglobulin |
| | Thyroid peroxidase |
| Graves' disease | TSH receptor |
| Pernicious anaemia | Intrinsic factor |
| | Parietal cell |
| Addison's disease | Adrenal cortex cells |
| Insulin-dependent diabetes mellitus | Cytoplasm of islet cells |
| | Insulin |
| | Glutamic acid decarboxylase (GAD) |
| Myasthenia gravis | Acetylcholine receptor |
| Lambert–Eaton syndrome | Calcium channels on nerve endings |
| Gullain–Barré syndrome | Peripheral nerve myelin components |
| Goodpasture's syndrome | Glomerular and lung basement membrane |
| Autoimmune haemolytic anaemia | Erythrocytes |
| Idiopathic thrombocytopenia | Platelets |
| Primary biliary cirrhosis | Mitochondria |
| Some male infertility | Spermatozoa |

Autoantibodies in rheumatological disorders – see Rheumatology.

## Some important HLA associations

**Table 25**

| HLA type | Disease |
| --- | --- |
| DR2 | Narcolepsy (100%) |
| | Multiple sclerosis |
| DR3 | Coeliac disease |
| | Dermatitis herpetiformis |
| | Type 1 diabetes |
| | Rheumatoid arthritis |
| | Systemic lupus erythematosus |
| | Graves' disease |
| | Addison's diseasae |
| DR4 | Rheumatoid arthritis |
| | Type 1 diabetes |
| A3 | Haemochromatosis |
| B27 | Ankylosing spondylitis |
| | Seronegative arthritides |

# Infectious Diseases

## Modes of transmission

1 Airborne, e.g. measles, diphtheria, tonsillitis, whooping cough, tuberculosis
2 Intestinal, e.g. enterovirus, viral hepatitis, poliomyelitis, salmonellosis
3 Direct contact, e.g. impetigo, scabies
4 Venereal route, e.g. gonorrhoea, syphilis
5 Insect or animal bite, e.g. malaria, leishmaniasis, trypanosomiasis, rabies
6 Blood borne, e.g. hepatitis B, HIV, hepatitis C
7 Congenital transmission.

## Factors affecting vulnerability to disease

1 Immunological:
   (a) Genetic deficiency – immunoglobulin/complement/T-cell deficiency
   (b) Prior immunity – natural or vaccine
   (c) Acquired deficiency – HIV, malignant disease, transplant patients
   (d) Miscellaneous – diabetes, pregnancy, splenectomy.
2 Other factors:
   (a) Psychological status
   (b) Nutritional status
   (c) Foreign bodies
   (d) Behavioural factors (smoking, alcoholism)
   (e) Previous antibiotics (e.g. *Clostridium difficile*, MRSA).

# Notifiable diseases (UK)

Anthrax
Cholera
Diphtheria
Dysentery (amoebic or bacillary)
Encephalitis
Food poisoning
Leprosy
Leptospirosis
Malaria
Measles
Meningitis
Meningococcal septicaemia
Mumps
Ophthalmia neonatorum
Plague
Poliomyelitis
Rabies
Relapsing fever
Rubella
Scarlet fever
Smallpox
Tetanus
Tuberculosis
Typhoid fever
Viral hepatitis
Viral haemorrhagic fever
Whooping cough
Yellow fever

# Definitions of sepsis

1  Systemic inflammatory response syndrome (SIRS) – defined as the presence of at least two of the following:
   (a)  Temperature $>38\,°C$ or $<36\,°C$
   (b)  Heart rate $>90$ bpm
   (c)  Respiratory rate $>20$/minute

(d) WCC $>12 \times 10^9/l$ or $<4 \times 10^9/l$

2 Sepsis: SIRS due to infective process, e.g. blood culture positive, abnormal CXR

3 Severe sepsis: sepsis with organ dysfunction (e.g. oliguria, confusion) or hypotension

4 Septic shock: hypotension despite fluid resuscitation or multi-organ failure.

Mortality rises significantly at each stage.

# Medically important Gram-positive bacteria

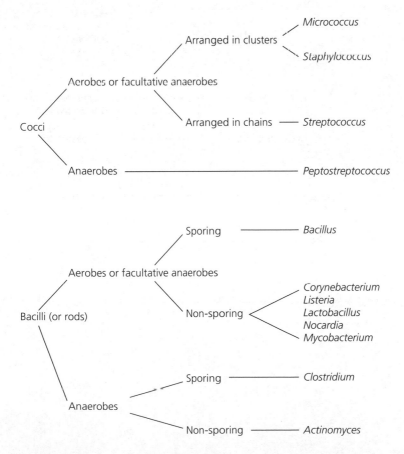

# Medically important Gram-negative bacteria

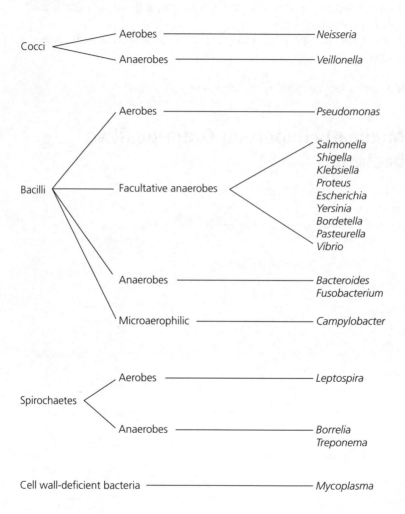

# Common travel illnesses

## Malaria

1 Caused by the protozoan *Plasmodium* species
2 Spread by the bite of the female *Anopheles* mosquito
3 There are four types:
  (a) Benign:
    (i) *P. vivax*
    (i) *P. ovale*
    (ii) *P. malariae*
  (b) Malignant – *P. falciparum*
4 Clinical features:
  (a) Fever with drenching sweats
  (b) Rigors
  (c) Headache
  (d) Myalgia
  (e) Diarrhoea and vomiting
5 Benign malaria is not life-threatening and is treated with chloroquine for three days followed by primaquine for two weeks (to eradicate liver cycle)
6 *Falciparum* malaria:
  (a) Complications:
    (i) Cerebral malaria (up to 10% mortality)
    (i) Haemolytic anaemia
    (ii) Metabolic acidosis
    (iii) Hypoglycaemia
    (iv) Acute renal failure
    (v) Pulmonary oedema
  (b) High parasite count = more severe disease
  (c) Treatment:
    (i) Oral or intravenous quinine
    (i) Alternatives include Malarone®, mefloquine
7 Diagnosis:
  (a) Serial thick and thin films
  (b) Rapid antigen tests
  (c) Other results:
    (i) Anaemia
    (ii) Thrombocytopenia

    (iii)  Hypoglycaemia
    (iv)  Abnormal coagulation
8  Remember always to consider malaria in a patient who has travelled to a malarious area even if they have taken prophylactic treatment.

## Dengue fever

1  Flavivirus infection
2  Spread by the daytime-biting *Aedes* mosquito
3  Clinical features:
    (a)  Fever
    (b)  Severe myalgia and bone pain (breakbone fever)
    (c)  Headache
    (d)  Nausea and vomiting
    (e)  Morbilliform rash
4  Usually a self-limiting illness
5  Can be complicated by dengue haemorrhagic fever (high mortality).

## Typhoid

1  *Salmonella typhi* infection
2  Faecal–oral transmission
3  Clinical features:
    (a)  Fever $>40\,°C$
    (b)  Headache
    (c)  Often constipation followed by diarrhoea
    (d)  Confusion
    (e)  Relative bradycardia
    (f)  Shock
    (g)  Rose spots on abdomen
    (h)  Hepatosplenomegaly
    (i)  Massive GI haemorrhage (bleeding Peyer's patches)
    (j)  Perforation of the bowel
4  Diagnosis:
    (a)  Blood culture
    (b)  Stool culture
    (c)  Serology
5  Treament of choice is ciprofloxacin
6  Untreated – 30% mortality
7  Vaccine only 70% protective.

# Viral infections

## Varicella zoster virus

1 Chickenpox is the primary infection
2 Transmitted by inhalation of virus
3 Characteristic crops of itchy vesicles, most pronounced on the trunk and head
4 Fever precedes rash by three days
5 Usually self-limiting but adults may develop more severe illness
6 Pneumonitis is a rare but severe complication (more common in smokers)
7 Chickenpox can cause life-threatening disease in immunocompromised patients
8 Treatment:
  (a) Symptomatic
  (b) Aciclovir can shorten illness if given within 48 hours of the rash
9 Shingles is the secondary form, caused by reactivation of virus from the dorsal root ganglion
10 Shingles develops in dematomes
11 Often causes very severe pain that can lasts for up to one year (post-herpetic neuralgia).

## Epstein–Barr virus (EBV)

1 Classically causes 'glandular fever'
2 Clinical features:
  (a) Sore throat
  (b) Fever
  (c) Headache
  (d) Lethargy
  (e) Generalised lymphadenopathy
  (f) Splenomegaly
  (g) Maculopapular rash if given penicillin
3 Diagnosis:
  (a) Abnormal lymphocytes on blood film
  (b) Monospot test
  (c) EBV serology
4 Other associated diseases:
  (a) Burkitt's lymphoma

(b) Hodgkin's lymphoma
(c) Lymphoma in AIDS patients
(d) Oral hairy leukoplakia.

# Sexually transmitted infections

1 Gonorrhoea:
   (a) Caused by *Neisseria gonorrhoea*
   (b) Transmission can be through oral/vaginal/anal intercourse
   (c) A large asymptomatic population
   (d) Symptoms include pus-like urethral discharge, itch, pain
   (e) Usually sensitive to penicillin
   (f) Left untreated → urethral strictures, pelvic inflammatory disease in women, prostatitis/epididymitis in men
   (g) Responsible for ophthalmia neonatorum
2 Chlamydial infection:
   (a) Caused by *Chlamydia trachomatis*
   (b) Responsible for over half of cases of non-specific urethritis (NSU), previously known as non-gonococcal urethritis (NGU)
   (c) A cause of pelvic inflammatory disease and infertility in women
   (d) Can cause conjunctivitis and a diffuse pneumonia in neonates
   (e) Sensitive to doxycycline and erythromycin
3 Trichomoniasis
   (a) Caused by a flagellated protozoan, *Trichomonas vaginalis*
   (b) Causes foul-smelling, greeny/yellow vaginal discharge and vaginitis
   (c) Treated with metronidazole
4 Herpes simplex virus (HSV):
   (a) Types 1 and 2
   (b) Can be dormant for very long periods of time
   (c) Leads to painful genital ulceration
   (d) Aciclovir helps reduce duration of lesions
   (e) Can recur after initial infection but normally less aggressively
5 Human papilloma virus (HPV):
   (a) Causes anogenital warts, benign tumours of the skin
   (b) Can cause large lesions around the anus, glans, labia or vagina, i.e. both skin and mucous membranes
   (c) Treated with cryotherapy and podophyllin

(d)  Often recur
(e)  Types 16 and 18 associated with carcinoma of the cervix
6  Syphilis:
(a)  Aetiological agent is *Treponema pallidum*
(b)  Transmission mainly sexual; incubation 2–4 weeks
(c)  Four clinical stages:
   (i)   Primary – painless genital ulceration, the classical chancre; heals in 3–8 weeks
   (ii)  Secondary – 6–8 weeks later the infection becomes generalised with rash, often papular
   (iii) Tertiary – 3–10 years after the primary lesion; gumma (granulomatous nodules) form in skin, mucous membranes or bones
   (iv)  Late or quarternary – 10–20 years after primary syphilis. There are two main forms, cardiovascular and neurological
(d)  Diagnosis is by direct demonstration of the spirochaete in the fluid of a chancre or ulcerated secondary lesion
(e)  There are three main serological tests for syphilis:
   (i)   The Venereal Disease Research Laboratory (VDRL) test
   (ii)  The *Treponema pallidum* haemagglutination assay (TPI IA)
   (iii) The fluorescent treponemal antibody (absorbed) test (FTA)
(f)  Treated with penicillin.

# Fungal infections

1  Aerobic organisms
2  Grow readily on simple media
3  Ubiquitous
4  Often a problem in immunocompromised patients
5  Can be divided into:
(a)  Yeasts
(b)  Filamentous fungi
(c)  Dimorphic fungi.

## Yeasts

1  *Candida albicans* – infects mucous membranes (thrush), may cause chronic mucocutaneous candidiasis. Can involve lower respiratory and urinary tracts, eye, meninges, kidney and bone

2 *Cryptococcus neoformans* – a lung granuloma is normally the subsequent primary focus, haematogenous spread leading to subacute or chronic meningoencephalitis.

### Filamentous fungi

1 Dermatophytes – ring worm/tinea. Affects nails, skin, hair
2 *Aspergillus* spp. – can cause a variety of clinical syndromes: allergic bronchopulmonary aspergillosis (ABPA), aspergilloma, invasive aspergillosis, superficial infections.

### Dimorphic fungi

1 Coccoidomycosis
2 Histoplasmosis
3 Blastomycosis.

# Causes of pyrexia of unknown origin (PUO)

1 Infection (35%):
   (a) TB
   (b) Hidden abscesses
   (c) Subacute bacterial endocarditis
   (d) Infectious mononucleosis
   (e) CMV
   (f) Brucellosis
   (g) Chronic prostatitis
2 Neoplasia (25%):
   (a) Hodgkin's disease and other lymphomas
   (b) Leukaemias
   (c) Solid tumours, e.g. renal, pancreatic, hepatocellular
   (d) Metastatic carcinoma
3 Connective tissue disease (20%):
   (a) Rheumatoid
   (b) SLE
   (c) Polyarteritis nodosa
4 Miscellaneous (15%):
   (a) Sarcoid

   (b) Multiple pulmonary emboli
   (c) Crohn's disease
   (d) Drugs
5 Undiagnosed (5–10%).

# Antimicrobial therapy

## Types of antibiotic

1 Inhibitors of cell wall synthesis:
   (a) Beta-lactams:
      (i)   Penicillins, e.g. benzyl penicillin, amoxicillin, piperacillin
      (ii)  Cephalosporins, e.g. cefalexin, cefotaxime
      (iii) Monobactams, e.g. aztreonam
      (iv) Carbapenems, e.g. imipenem
   (b) Glycopeptides – vancomycin, teicoplanin
2 Inhibitors of protein synthesis:
   (a) Macrolides – erythromycin, clarithromycin
   (b) Aminoglycosides – gentamicin, tobramycin
   (c) Tetracycline
   (d) Miscellaneous:
      (i)   Chloramphenicol
      (ii)  Clindamycin
      (iii) Fusidic acid
3 Inhibitors of DNA replication:
   (a) Quinolones, e.g. ciprofloxacin
   (b) Metronidazole
4 Inhibitors of folate synthesis:
   (a) Trimethoprim
   (b) Co-trimoxazole.

## Antituberculous drugs

1 Rifampicin – inhibits DNA-dependent RNA polymerase
2 Isoniazid – inhibits cell wall synthesis
3 Pyrazinamide – poorly understood, probably works inside phagosomes
4 Ethambutol – inhibits bacterial RNA synthesis
5 Streptomycin – inhibits bacterial protein synthesis.

## Antiviral drugs (non-HIV)

1  Aciclovir – active against HSV and VZV
2  Ganciclovir – as above but also against CMV
3  Ribavirin – used against HCV, RSV, Lassa fever (has to be early).

## Antifungal drugs

1  Nystatin – *Candida*
2  Fluconazole – *Candida*, *Cryptococcus*
3  Itraconazole – *Candida*, *Aspergillus*
4  Amphotericin – *Aspergillus*, serious invasive fungal infections
5  Flucytosine – used in combination for cryptococcal infections.

# Metabolic Medicine

## Lipids

### Hyperlipidaemias

1 Atherosclerotic disease associated with high total cholesterol and LDL
2 HDL is protective.

### *Primary disorders*

1 Familial hypercholesterolaemia:
   (a) Autosomal dominant; heterozygotes 1 in 500
   (b) Defect in LDL receptor
   (c) Total cholesterol 9–15 mmol/l
   (d) Six to eight times increased risk of IHD (MI at young age)
   (e) Other features are xanthelasma and tendon xanthomata
   (f) Treat with diet and statins
2 Familial triglyceridaemia:
   (a) Autosomal dominant
   (b) Associated with eruptive xanthomata, pancreatitis, retinal vein thrombosis, hepatosplenomegaly, lipaemia retinalis
   (c) Treat with diet and fibrates
3 Lipoprotein lipase deficiency:
   (a) Rare
   (b) Failure to break down chylomicrons
4 Familial combined hyperlipidaemia:
   (a) Elevated cholesterol and triglycerides
   (b) Main feature is atherosclerosis.

*Causes of secondary hyperlipidaemia*

1 Mainly raised cholesterol:
   (a) Hypothyroidism
   (b) Cholestasis
   (c) Nephrotic syndrome
   (d) Renal transplant
2 Mainly raised triglycerides:
   (a) Obesity
   (b) Chronic alcohol excess
   (c) Insulin resistance and diabetes
   (d) Chronic liver disease
   (e) Thiazide diuretics
   (f) High-dose oestrogens.

# Sodium

## Causes of hypernatraemia

1 Fluid loss without water replacement (burns, vomiting)
2 Excessive fluid replacement with saline
3 Conn's syndrome
4 Diabetes insipidus
5 Diabetic ketoacidosis
6 Hyperosmolar non-ketotic state (HONK).

## Causes of hyponatraemia

### *Patient dehydrated*

1 Diuretic excess
2 Addison's disease
3 Renal failure (diuretic phase)
4 Pseudohyponatraemia (DKA).

### *Patient well hydrated*

1 Syndrome of inappropriate ADH secretion (SIADH)
2 Nephrotic syndrome
3 Congestive cardiac failure

4 Liver cirrhosis
5 Renal failure
6 Water overload
7 Hypothyroidism
8 Pseudohyponatraemia (hyperlipidaemia).

## Causes of syndrome of inappropriate ADH secretion (SIADH)

1 Malignancy:
   (a) Bronchus, bladder, prostate, pancreas
   (b) Lymphoma
   (c) Mesothelioma
2 Pulmonary disorders:
   (a) Pneumonia
   (b) Abscess
   (c) TB
   (d) Asthma
3 Neurological:
   (a) Encephalitis and meningitis
   (b) Trauma
   (c) Acute intermittent porphyria
   (d) Guillain–Barré syndrome
   (e) Subarachnoid haemorrhage
   (f) Hydrocephalus
   (g) Acute psychosis
4 Drugs:
   (a) Chlorpropamide
   (b) Carbamazepine
   (c) Tolbutamide.

## Diabetes insipidus

1 Cranial causes (altered production ± secretion of ADH):
   (a) Idiopathic
   (b) Craniopharyngioma
   (c) Infiltrative processes of the hypothalamus, e.g. sarcoidosis
   (d) Trauma
   (e) Pituitary surgery
2 Nephrogenic causes (decreased action of ADH):
   (a) Primary – X-linked/dominant tubular receptor abnormality

   (b) Secondary:
      (i)  Hypercalcaemia
      (ii)  Hypokalaemia
      (iii) Renal disease: chronic pyelonephritis, adult polycystic kidney disease, post-obstruction
      (iv) Drugs: lithium, demeclocycline.

# Potassium

## Hyperkalaemia

### Causes

1 Spurious:
   (a)  Haemolysis
   (b)  Delayed separation of serum
   (c)  Contamination
2 Excessive intake:
   (a)  Oral (uncommon)
   (b)  Parenteral
3 Decreased excretion:
   (a)  Acute oliguric renal failure
   (b)  Chronic renal failure
   (c)  Potassium-sparing diuretics
   (d)  ACE inhibitors
   (e)  Mineralocorticoid deficiency (Addison's disease)
4 Redistribution:
   (a)  Tissue damage, e.g. rhabdomyolysis
   (b)  Acidosis, particularly DKA
   (c)  Catabolic states.

### ECG changes

1 Tenting of T waves
2 Reduction in size of P waves
3 Increase in PR interval
4 Widening QRS complexes.

## *Treatment*

1  Intravenous calcium gluconate 10%
2  Intravenous insulin and dextrose
3  Calcium resonium®
4  Furosemide (frusemide)
5  Salbutamol nebulisers
6  Dialysis.

## Causes of hypokalaemia

1  Decreased intake:
   (a)  Oral (uncommon except in starvation)
   (b)  Parenteral
2  Increased excretion:
   (a)  Gastrointestinal:
      (i)  Diarrhoea
      (ii)  Vomiting
      (iii)  Purgative abuse
      (iv)  Villous adenoma
   (b)  Renal:
      (i)  Diuretics – loops and thiazides
      (ii)  Diuretic phase of acute renal failure
      (iii)  Renal tubular acidosis
   (c)  Endocrine:
      (i)  Cushing's syndrome
      (ii)  Mineralocorticoid excess, e.g. steroids, liquorice
   (d)  Redistribution:
      (i)  Insulin, alkalosis
      (ii)  Rapid cellular proliferation.

# Bone and minerals

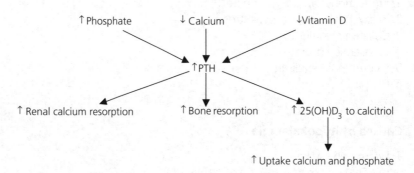

### Vitamin D

1 Mostly made in skin by action of UV light
2 25-hydroxylated in the liver
3 Hydroxylated again to $1,25(OH)_2D_3$ (calcitriol) in the kidney.

### Hypercalcaemia

#### Causes

1 Primary hyperparathyroidism (adenoma of parathyroid gland)
2 Malignancy (PTH-related protein and bone metastases)
3 ↑ Calcium intake (and milk-alkali syndrome)
4 ↑ Vitamin D
5 Tertiary hyperparathyroidism
6 Hyperthyroidism
7 Sarcoid (macrophages in lesions produce $1,25(OH)_2D_3$
8 Thiazides.

#### Features

1 As underlying condition, plus
2 Lethargy, malaise and depression
3 Weakness
4 Confusion
5 Constipation
6 Nausea
7 Renal stones

8 Diabetes insipidus (polyuria, polydipsia)
9 Pancreatitis.

## Treatment

1 Aggressive rehydration
2 Intravenous diphosphonate (pamidronate).

## Hyperparathyroidism

1 Primary:
  (a) Single adenoma in $> 80\%$
  (b) Carcinoma very rare
  (c) Results in ↑ PTH, ↑ serum and urinary calcium, ↑ alkaline phosphatase and ↓ serum phosphate
  (d) Causes increased osteoblast and osteoclast activity, therefore bone turnover (bone loss can occur)
2 Secondary – due to hypertrophy of glands in response to chronic hypocalcaemia (e.g. in renal failure)
3 Tertiary – consequence of long-standing secondary hyperparathyroidism. Further gland hyperplasia raises calcium levels
4 Treatment is parathyroidectomy.

## Hypocalcaemia

### Causes

1 Hypoparathyroidism
2 Low levels of vitamin $D_3$ (diet, malabsorption)
3 Hyperphosphataemia (chronic renal failure)
4 Hypomagnesaemia
5 Sepsis
6 Respiratory alkalosis
7 Calcium deposition (pancreatitis).

### Features

1 Muscle weakness
2 Neuromuscular excitability
3 Confusion
4 Seizures
5 Tetany

  6 Alopecia
  7 Brittle nails
  8 Cataracts
  9 Dental hypoplasia
10 Osteomalacia/rickets.

## Treatment

Supplementation of calcium, vitamin $D_3$.

## Causes of hypoparathyroidism

1 Parathyroidectomy (intentional or accidental)
2 Autoimmune
3 Receptor defect (pseudohypoparathyroidism)

## Osteomalacia/rickets

Decreased mineralisation of osteoid.

## Causes

1 Vitamin D deficiency (diet, malabsorption)
2 Impaired calcium metabolism
3 Renal failure
4 Chronic liver disease.

## Clinical features

1 Pain
2 Deformity (bow legs, abnormal ribs and skull)
3 Fractures
4 Proximal myopathy
5 Raised alkaline phosphatase.

## Paget's disease

1 Increased bone turnover with abnormal new bone turnover
2 Causes pain, deformity, arthritis, nerve compression, fractures, sarcoma
3 Associated with greatly raised alkaline phosphatase. Calcium only raised with immobility

4 Treatment: analgesia, bisphosphonates.

## Osteoporosis

1 Reduced bone mass and density
2 Abnormal bone microarchitecture.

### Primary

1 Type I: oestrogen deficiency post-menopause. Affects mainly trabecular bone
2 Type II: age-related decrease in osteoblastic activity. Affects cortical and trabecular bone.

### Secondary

1 Drugs: steroids, heparin
2 Endocrine: Cushing's, hyperparathyroidism, premature menopause, hyperthyroidism, hypogonadism
3 Malignancy: myeloma, leukaemia
4 Gastrointestinal: malabsorption syndromes, primary biliary cirrhosis
5 Inflammatory disorders: inflammatory bowel disease, RA
6 Immobilisation: non-weight-bearing (space flight)
7 Miscellaneous: alcoholism, smoking, Turner's syndrome.

### Tests

1 Calcium, phosphate, alkaline phosphatase normal
2 Diagnosis by DEXA scan.

### Treatment

1 Treatment of any secondary cause
2 Hormone replacement therapy
3 Calcium and vitamin D
4 Calcitonin
5 Bisphosphonates.

### Interpretation of results in patients with bone disease

**Table 26**

| Disease | Ca | PO4 | ALP | PTH |
|---|---|---|---|---|
| Hyperparathyroidism (primary) | ↑ | ↓ or N | ↑ or N | ↑ |
| Hypoparathyroidism | ↓ | ↑ | N | ↓ |
| Osteoporosis | N | N | N | N |
| Osteomalacia | ↓ | ↓ | ↑ | ↑ |
| Paget's disease | N | N | ↑↑ | N |
| Renal failure | ↓ | ↑ | ↑ or N | ↑ |

# Copper

1  50% of ingested copper is absorbed
2  Binds with globulin to form caeruloplasmin.

### Wilson's disease

1  Autosomal recessive
2  Abnormality of caeruloplasmin formation leading to accumulation of copper in the body
3  Features: acute/chronic hepatitis, cirrhosis, Kayser–Fleischer rings, CNS symptoms, arthropathy
4  Diagnosis: low caeruloplasmin, high urinary copper, liver biopsy
5  Treatment: penicillamine (copper chelator), liver transplant.

# Iron

1  There is 4 g in the normal human body, two-thirds in haemoglobin
2  There is 20 mg per day in a normal diet; only 10% absorbed
3  $Fe^{2+}$ more readily absorbed than $Fe^{3+}$
4  Transferrin normally one-third saturated
5  Ferritin (acute phase protein) increased in iron overload, decreased in deficiency
6  Plasma iron levels show great variation.

## Haemochromatosis

1 Autosomal recessive
2 Commoner, more severe in men (no menstruation)
3 Features: micronodular cirrhosis, chondrocalcinosis, pseudogout, skin bronzing, diabetes, cardiomyopathy, arrhythmias
4 Diagnosis: raised serum iron and ferritin. Transferrin >60% saturated. HFE gene testing. Liver biopsy
5 Most common cause of secondary iron overload is multiple transfusions
6 Treatment: venesection, desferrioxamine.

# Acid–base disorders

## Metabolic acidosis

1 Increased anion gap:
  (a) Lactic acidosis (sepsis, hypoxia, metformin)
  (b) Renal failure
  (c) Diabetic ketocidosis
  (d) Drugs – ethylene glycol, salicylates
2 Normal ion gap:
  (a) Renal tubular acidosis
  (b) Diarrhoea
  (c) Addison's disease.

## Metabolic alkalosis

1 Vomiting
2 Hypokalaemia
3 Burns
4 Ingestion of base.

## Respiratory acidosis

Hypoventilation.

## Respiratory alkalosis

Hyperventilation.

# Deficiencies

## Protein–energy malnutrition

1 Undernutrition – weight 60–80% of standard for age, no oedema
2 Marasmus:
   (a) Deficient in protein and calories
   (b) Weight < 60% of standard, no oedema
3 Kwashiorkor:
   (a) Solely due to protein deficiency
   (b) Weight 60–80% of standard, oedema present
   (c) Fatty liver often seen.

## Vitamin deficiencies

**Table 27**

| Vitamin | Cause of deficiency | Consequence of deficiency |
|---|---|---|
| A | Protein–energy malnutrition | Night blindness, dry corneas, keratomalacia |
| B$_1$ (thiamine) | Alcoholism, dietary restriction | Dry beri-beri: Wernicke–Korsakoff, polyneuropathy Wet beri-beri: high-output cardiac failure |
| B$_2$ (riboflavin) | Protein-energy malnutrition | Glossitis, angular stomatitis |
| Niacin | Alcoholism, isoniazid, carcinoid syndrome | Pellagra – **d**ermatitis, **d**iarrhoea, **d**ementia and **d**eath |
| B$_6$ (pyridoxine) | Hydralazine, isoniazid | Peripheral neuropathy, glossitis |
| B$_{12}$ (cyanocobalamin) | Pernicious anaemia, gastrectomy, ileal disease, vegans | Macrocytic anaemia, subacute combined degeneration of the cord |
| C | Dietary deficiency | Scurvy: gingivitis, bleeding, joint swelling |
| D | Renal failure, dietary | Osteomalacia, rickets |
| E | Fat malabsorption, abetalipoproteinaemia | Spinocerebellar degeneration |
| K | Biliary obstruction, antibiotic therapy | Bleeding diathesis |

# Tumour markers

| | |
|---|---|
| AFP | Hepatocellular carcinoma, germ cell tumours |
| CA125 | Ovarian cancer, breast cancer |
| CEA | Colorectal carcinoma |
| HCG | Germ cell tumours |
| PSA | Prostate carcinoma. |

# Interpretation of biochemical results

Causes of raised plasma enzymes:

| | |
|---|---|
| ALP | Liver disease (cholestasis) |
| | Bone disease (osteoblast activity) |
| | Pregnancy |
| ALT | Hepatocellular damage |
| AST | Hepatocellular damage |
| | MI (peak 48 hours) |
| | Muscle damage |
| | Haemolysis |
| Amylase | Acute pancreatitis |
| CK | MI |
| | Muscle damage |
| | Hypothyroidism |
| | Drugs (statins) |
| GGT | Liver disease (cholestasis and alcohol-related liver disease) |
| Ferritin | Acute phase response |
| | Haemochromatosis |
| | Iron therapy |
| | Thalassaemia |
| LDH | Liver disease |
| | MI (peak 72 hours) |
| | Haemolysis |

# Nephrology

## Symptoms and signs in renal disease

### Clinical features of uraemia

1 Neurological:
   (a) Malaise
   (b) Depression
   (c) Fits
   (d) Coma
2 Cardiorespiratory:
   (a) Pericarditis
   (b) Pleurisy
   (c) Kussmaul breathing (acidosis)
3 Dermatological:
   (a) Pruritis
   (b) Purpura (abnormal platelet function)
   (c) Pigmentation
4 Gastrointestinal:
   (a) Anorexia
   (b) Nausea and vomiting
   (c) Gastrointestinal bleeding
   (d) Diarrhoea
   (e) Constipation.

### Causes of proteinuria

1 Infection:
   (a) Fever
   (b) Urinary tract infection
   (c) Chronic pyelonephritis
   (d) Renal TB
2 Glomerular disease:
   (a) Acute and chronic glomerulonephritis
   (b) Diabetes

   (c)  Hypertension (including pre-eclampsia)
3 Neoplastic:
   (a)  Renal tract tumour
   (b)  Myeloma
4 Other causes:
   (a)  Interstitial nephritis
   (b)  Acute tubular necrosis (ATN).

## Causes of urinary frequency

1 Infection:
   (a)  Cystitis
   (b)  Urethritis
   (c)  Prostatitis
2 Bladder tumour
3 Prostatic hypertrophy
4 Urethral stricture
5 Neurological, e.g. multiple sclerosis.

## Causes of coloured urine

1 Haematuria
2 Haemoglobinuria
3 Drugs, e.g. rifampicin
4 Beetroot
5 Myoglobinuria
6 Obstructive jaundice
7 Porphyria.

## Causes of macroscopic haematuria

1 Urinary tract malignancy
2 Urinary infections
3 Acute glomerulonephritis
4 IgA nephropathy
5 Renal calculi
6 Renal papillary necrosis
7 Prostatic hypertrophy
8 Trauma.

# Investigations

## Creatinine

1 Raised creatinine:
   (a) Renal impairment
   (b) Large muscle bulk
   (c) Rhabdomyolysis
   (d) Decreased tubular secretion, e.g. trimethoprim, K-sparing diuretics
2 Reduced creatinine:
   (a) Small muscle mass
   (b) Pregnancy
   (c) Raised ADH.

## Urea

1 Raised urea:
   (a) Reduced glomerular filtration rate (GFR), e.g. dehydration
   (b) Gastrointestinal bleeding
   (c) Corticosteroids/tetracycline
   (d) High protein diet
   (e) Increased catabolism
2 Reduced urea:
   (a) Liver disease, e.g. excess alcohol
   (b) Starvation/anabolic state
   (c) Raised ADH
   (d) Pregnancy.

# Acute renal failure

## Causes

Over 90% are due to prerenal causes or acute tubular necrosis.
1 Prerenal – appropriate renal response to poor renal perfusion
2 Renal:
   (a) Acute tubular necrosis
      (i) Following circulatory compromise (hypovolaemia, haemorrhage)

      (ii)  Sepsis

      (iii)  Following nephrotoxins (drugs, toxins)

      (iv)  Often multiple causes

(b)  Vascular causes:

      (i)  Large vessel occlusion, e.g. renal artery stenosis or thrombosis

      (ii)  Accelerated hypertension

      (iii)  Scleroderma

      (iv)  Pre-eclampsia

(c)  Glomerulonephritis (GN):

      (i)  Primary GN:
- Mesangial IgA nephropathy
- Mesangiocapillary GN

      (ii)  Infection-related GN:
- Post-infection (streptococcal)
- Infective endocarditis
- Others, e.g. abscesses

(d)  Interstitial nephritis:

      (i)  Drugs:
- Antibiotics, e.g. penicillins, rifampicin, sulphonamides
- NSAIDs
- Diuretics, e.g. thiazides, furosemide (frusemide)

      (ii)  Infection-related:
- UTI, pyelonephritis
- *Legionella*
- Epstein–Barr virus
- Leptospiral infection

(e)  Vasculitis:

      (i)  Goodpasture's syndrome

      (ii)  Wegener's granulomatosis

      (iii)  Microscopic polyangiitis

      (iv)  Churg–Strauss syndrome

      (v)  Henoch–Schönlein purpura

      (vi)  Cryoglobulinaemia

(f)  Haematological:

      (i)  Myeloma

      (ii)  Haemolytic uraemic syndrome

(g)  Other causes:

      (i)  Rhabdomyolysis

      (ii)  Hepatorenal syndrome

      (iii)  SLE

(iv)  Pancreatitis
(v)   Electrolyte disturbance, e.g. hypercalcaemia
(vi)  Urate nephropathy
3  Postrenal – urinary obstruction:
   (a)  Renal stones
   (b)  Benign and malignant obstructive lesions of the renal tract or
        prostate
   (c)  Retroperitoneal fibrosis
   (d)  Papillary necrosis.

## Acute tubular necrosis (ATN)

1  Ischaemic damage due to renal hypoperfusion (hypovolaemia, sepsis
   etc.)
2  Reversible in time but time taken varies (may need dialysis until
   recovery occurs)
3  Initial treatment requires aggressive fluid resuscitation but urine
   output remains low.

It is important to distinguish between ATN and prerenal uraemia:
1  Prerenal uraemia produces low-volume concentrated urine
2  ATN gives low- or high-volume, dilute, 'poor quality' urine
3  Prerenal failure responds quickly to fluid resuscitation with an increase
   in urine output.

## Serious complications of ARF

1  Hyperkalaemia (see Metabolic Medicine)
2  Pulmonary oedema
3  Intravascular volume depletion/overload
4  Bleeding.

## Investigation of ARF

1  Full history and examination:
   (a)  ? Systemic cause
   (b)  Drug history – penicillin or NSAIDs
2  Ultrasound scan:
   (a)  Rule out obstruction
   (b)  Kidney size (if small then acute on chronic)
3  Urine testing:

(a)  Microscopy of urine (cells, casts, crystals)
(b)  Stix and biochemical tests (protein, glucose, specific gravity)
(c)  Culture and sensitivity
(d)  Bence Jones protein
4  IVU (Intravenous urogram)
5  Isotope renography:
(a)  Static, e.g. DMSA
(b)  Dynamic, e.g. MAG3, DTPA
(c)  Captopril renogram to look for renovascular disease
6  Specific blood tests:
(a)  Anti-GBM antibodies – Goodpasture's syndrome
(b)  ANCA – systemic vasculitis
(c)  Anti-dsDNA and anti-Sm – SLE
(d)  ASOT – poststreptococcal glomerulonephritis
(e)  Blood cultures – infection-related, especially endocarditis
7  Less specific blood tests:
(a)  Complement
(b)  Immunoglobulins:
   (i)   Monoclonal increase in myeloma
   (ii)  Raised IgE in Churg–Strauss syndrome
   (iii) Raised IgA in Henoch–Schölein purpura and IgA nephropathy
(c)  Cryoglobulins – cryoglobulinaemia
(d)  CRP – increased in most cases but not usually in SLE
(e)  Neutrophilia, thrombocytosis – systemic vasculitis
(f)  Eosinophilia:
   (i)   Drug-induced interstitial nephritis
   (ii)  Churg–Strauss syndrome
(g)  Lymphopenia – SLE
(h)  Thrombocytopenia – drug-induced interstitial nephritis, SLE.

## Criteria for urgent dialysis

1  Severe hyperkalaemia
2  Fluid overload leading to pulmonary oedema
3  Acidosis resulting in circulatory compromise
4  Uraemia causing encephalopathy, pericarditis or bleeding.

## Rhabdomyolysis

1  Muscle damage or necrosis leading to myoglobin release

2  Clinical features:
   (a)  ARF
   (b)  Raised potassium and phosphate
   (c)  Creatine kinase massively raised
   (d)  Creatinine raised disproportionately to urea
3  Causes:
   (a)  Trauma/compression injury
   (b)  Uncontrolled fitting
   (c)  Statins
   (d)  Burns.

# Chronic renal failure

## Causes (UK)

1  Diabetes mellitus 20%
2  Chronic glomerulonephritis 20%
3  Renovascular (including hypertension) 15%
4  Chronic reflux nephropathy 15%
5  Polycystic kidney disease 10%
6  Postobstructive 10%
7  Myeloma 3%
8  Amyloidosis 3%
9  Chronic interstitial nephritis
10  Analgesic nephropathy
11  Renal calculi
12  Post-acute renal failure.

## Management of chronic renal disease

1  Blood pressure control (aim for < 130/80 mmHg):
   (a)  ACE inhibitors
   (b)  Other antihypertensives
   (c)  Diuretics
2  Reduction in proteinuria – ACE inhibitors
3  Treatment of anaemia (maintain > 10 g/dl):
   (a)  Intravenous iron
   (b)  Erythropoietin
4  Diet:

(a) Low salt intake
(b) Low potassium intake
(c) High calorie intake
5 Treatment of hyperphosphataemia and hypocalcaemia (renal bone disease):
(a) Phosphate binders
(b) Alphacalcidol
6 Glucose control in diabetics
7 Hyperlipidaemia control
8 Volume status monitoring
9 Avoid nephrotoxic drugs.

## Anaemia of chronic renal failure

1 Occurs at GFR < 35 ml/minute
2 Due to lack of erythropoietin (normally produced by the kidneys)
3 Management:
(a) Subcutaneous erythropoietin (EPO) injections
(b) If ferritin < 100 $\mu$g/l then give intravenous iron.

## Renal osteodystrophy

1 Bone disease that results from the metabolic disturbance in renal failure
2 Causative factors:
(a) Low plasma ionised calcium, due to:
(i) Lack of 1,25(OH)$_2$ vitamin D
(ii) Malabsorption of calcium
(b) Hyperphosphataemia (failure of excretion)
(c) Stimulation of parathyroid hormone release (secondary hyperparathyroidism), due to:
(i) Hypocalcaemia
(ii) Hyperphosphataemia
(iii) Low 1,25(OH)$_2$ vitamin D
(iv) Acidosis
3 Clinical features:
(a) Osteoporosis
(b) Osteomalacia
(c) Areas of osteosclerosis (rugger-jersey spine)
4 Treatment:

(a) Phosphate binders (e.g. calcium acetate)
(b) Vitamin D (1-alphacalcidol)
(c) Parathyroidectomy.

## Renal transplantation

1 2000 patients per year in the UK
2 Graft survival: 90% at one year; 70% at five years
3 Live donors: 10–15% of transplants.

### Post-transplant complications

1 Rejection (see Immunology)
2 Malignancy:
    (a) Non-Hodgkin's lymphoma (especially ciclosporin)
    (b) Skin cancer (especially azathioprine)
3 Cardiovascular – IHD 10–20 times more prevalent
4 Hypertension in >50%
5 Infections:
    (a) Opportunistic, e.g. PCP, CMV
    (b) Myocarditis
    (c) Encephalitis
    (d) Retinitis
    (e) May lead to deterioration of renal function
6 Recurrence of disease after transplant (all glomerulonephritides can recur).

# Glomerulonephritis (GN)

## Definitions

1 Asymptomatic proteinuria: < 3 g/day
2 Nephrotic syndrome: > 3 g/day, oedema, serum albumin <25 g/l and increased cholesterol
3 Nephritic syndrome: hypertension, haematuria, oedema and oliguria
4 Haematuria: microscopic or macroscopic.

## Causes of nephrotic syndrome

1 Glomerulonephritis

2  Diabetes mellitus
3  Infection:
   (a)  Malaria
   (b)  Leprosy
   (c)  Hepatitis B
4  Pre-eclampsia
5  Accelerated hypertension
6  Myeloma
7  Amyloidosis
8  SLE
9  Drugs:
   (a)  Gold
   (b)  Penicillamine
   (c)  Captopril
   (d)  NSAIDs.

## Types of glomerulonephritis

1  Minimal-change GN:
   (a)  Commonest
   (b)  Presents with nephrotic syndrome
   (c)  Good prognosis
2  Membranous GN
3  Focal segmental glomerulosclerosis (FSGS)
4  Mesangioproliferative GN (IgA nephropathy or Berger's disease):
   presents with macroscopic haematuria, usually following pharyngitis
5  Mesangiocapillary GN
6  Diffuse proliferative GN: causes include poststreptococcal infection
7  Rapidly progressive GN (crescentic):
   (a)  Severe and rapidly progresses to end-stage renal failure (ESRF) in
        weeks to months
   (b)  Causes include Wegener's granulomatosis, Goodpasture's
        syndrome and SLE
   (c)  Treatment with high-dose steroids and immunosuppressives
   (d)  Often require dialysis and transplantation.

## Goodpasture's syndrome

1  Autoantibody to glomerular basement membrane (anti-GBM)
2  Pathology:

(a)  Rapidly progressive GN
(b)  Pulmonary haemorrhage
3  Presents with:
  (a)  Haemoptysis
  (b)  Haematuria
  (c)  Breathlessness
  (d)  Massive pulmonary haemorrhage
4  Management:
  (a)  Steroids
  (b)  Cyclophosphamide
  (c)  Plasma exchange
5  Prognosis: depends on renal function at presentation.

Other vasculitides see Rheumatology.

# Polycystic kidney disease

1  Autosomal dominant inheritance
2  Multiple renal cysts develop in teenage years
3  Presents with:
  (a)  Abdominal pain
  (b)  Haematuria
  (c)  Urinary tract infection
  (d)  Hypertension
  (e)  Renal failure
4  Associations:
  (a)  Liver cysts and/or pancreatic cysts
  (b)  Berry aneurysms
  (c)  Malignant change
  (d)  Mitral valve prolapse.

## Acute interstitial nephritis

1  Inflammatory condition of renal interstitium
2  Presents with:
  (a)  Mild renal impairment
  (b)  Hypertension
  (c)  Interstitial oedema on biopsy with acute tubular necrosis
3  Causes (above)

4 Treatment:
   (a) Remove the cause, e.g. drug
   (b) Some require small dose of steroids
5 Most make a complete recovery.


# Renal calculi

1 Prevalence 3% in the UK
2 Calcium-containing caculi are the most common
3 Predisposing factors:
   (a) Metabolic:
       (i)   Hypercalciuria
       (ii)  Primary hypercalcaemia
       (iii) Renal tubular acidosis
       (iv)  Uric aciduria
       (v)   Hyperoxaluria
   (b) Structural:
       (i)   Polcystic kidney disease
       (ii)  Reflux nephropathy
       (iii) Nephrocalcinosis
       (iv)  Medullary sponge kidney
   (c) Others – dehydration
4 Clinical features:
   (a) May be asymptomatic
   (b) Renal colic
   (c) Haematuria
   (d) Proteinuria
   (e) Cystitis
   (f) Pyelonephritis
   (g) Pyonephrosis
   (h) Obstruction
5 Treatment:
   (a) Increase fluid intake
   (b) Reduce calcium or oxalate intake
   (c) Treat underlying cause
   (d) Thiazide diuretic (reduces hypercalciuria)
   (e) Stone removal and/or lithotripsy.

# Systemic disorders and the kidney

## Amyloidosis

1 Chronic infiltrative disorders that leads to deposition of amyloid proteins in tissues
2 Classification:
   (a) Primary amyloid (AL)
   (b) Secondary amyloid (AA or AL)
   (c) Senile amyloid (pre-albumin)
   (d) Dialysis amyloid ($\beta_2$ microglobulin)
3 Clinical features:
   (a) Proteinuria (asymptomatic to nephrotic)
   (b) Chronic renal failure
   (c) Hepatosplenomegaly
   (d) Macroglossia
   (e) Malabsorption
   (f) Restrictive cardiomyopathy
4 Diagnosis by histology: Congo red stain on biopsy
5 Causes of secondary amyloidosis (mainly chronic inflammatory conditions):
   (a) Rheumatoid conditions (RA, seronegative arthritis, scleroderma)
   (b) Inflammatory bowel disease
   (c) Tuberculosis
   (d) Osteomyelitis
   (e) Bronchiectasis
   (f) Myeloma.

## Renovascular disease

1 Associated with general vascular disease
2 Co-morbidity high and therefore poor prognosis
3 Presents with:
   (a) Hypertension
   (b) Flash pulmonary oedema
   (c) End-stage renal failure
   (d) Chronic renal failure
   (e) Acute renal failure following ACE inhibitor or angiotensin-II antagonist
4 Investigations:

(a)  Asymmetrical kidneys on ultrasound scan
(b)  Captopril renogram
(c)  Magnetic resonance angiogram
(d)  Conventional angiography
5  Treatment:
(a)  Angioplasty ± stenting
(b)  Aspirin
(c)  Antihypertensives
(d)  Lipid-lowering treatment.

## Diabetes mellitus (DM)

1  Most common cause of ESRF in the UK
2  Renal disease present in 49% of type 1 diabetics 20–40 years from diagnosis of DM
3  Presents with:
(a)  Microalbuminuria (30–250 mg/day)
(b)  Proteinuria ( > 0.5 g/day)
(c)  Hypertension
(d)  Nephrotic syndrome
(e)  Chronic renal failure
4  Kimmelstiel–Wilson nodules are characteristic on renal biopsy
5  Treatment:
(a)  ACE inhibitors and angiotensin blockers
(b)  Tight glycaemic control
(c)  Tight blood pressure control (target is < 130/75 mmHg).

## Connective tissue disorders

### SLE nephritis

1  40% of SLE patients have renal involvement
2  Any presentation possible
3  Histology variable
4  Treatment:
(a)  ARF and SLE – aggressive immunosuppressant therapy
(b)  Maintenance with oral steroids and azathioprine
(c)  Plasma exchange.

### *Systemic sclerosis*

1 Presents with:
  (a) Accelerated hypertension
  (b) Micro-angiopathic haemolytic anaemia (MAHA)
  (c) Acute renal failure
2 Histology: onion-skin appearance of interlobular arteries
3 Treatment: ACE inhibitor for hypertension
4 Many progress to end-stage renal failure.

# Nephrotoxic drugs

See Clinical Pharmacology.

# Tumours of the renal tract

1 Benign:
  (a) Adenoma
  (b) Hamartoma
  (c) Renin-secreting (juxtaglomerular cell) – leads to Conn's syndrome
2 Renal cell carcinoma:
  (a) Arises from tubular epithelium
  (b) Clinical features:
     (i) Haematuria
     (ii) Loin pain
     (iii) Abdominal mass
     (iv) PUO
     (v) Renal vein invasion
     (vi) Left testicular vein occlusion leads to left-sided varicocele
     (vii) Polycythaemia – excess erythropoietin production
     (viii) Hypertension (renin secretion)
3 Wilms' Tumour: tumour of embryonic tissue in children
4 Urothelial tumours:
  (a) Transitional cell origin
  (b) Commonly present with bleeding or urinary tract obstruction
  (c) Often multiple
  (d) Risk factors:
     (i) Smoking

(ii)   Analgesic nephropathy
(iii)  Exposure to rubber or aniline dyes
(iv)  Renal calculi
(v)   *Schistosoma* infection.

# Urinary tract infections (UTI)

## Causes

1  *Escherichia coli*: 60–90%
2  *Proteus mirabilis*: 10%
3  *Staphylococcus saprophyticus*: an important cause in sexually active women
4  *Klebsiella* spp.
5  *Streptococcus faecalis*
6  'Fastidious' Gram-positive bacteria: *Lactobacillus*, streptococci, corynebacteria
7  Organisms after catheterisation: e.g. *Pseudomonas aeruginosa*, *S. aureus*
8  *Mycobacterium tuberculosis*.

## Causes of sterile pyuria

1  Recently treated UTI
2  TB
3  Acute interstitial nephritis
4  Chronic interstitial nephritis
5  Chronic pyelonephritis.

# Neurology

## Interpreting cerebral lesions

### The cerebral cortex

Motor – precentral gyrus (frontal lobe).
Sensory
1  Somatosensory – postcentral gyrus
2  Auditory – superior temporal lobe
3  Visual – occipital cortex
4  Olfactory – frontal lobe
5  Broca's area – dominant frontal lobe, speech output
6  Wernicke's area – dominant posterior superior temporal gyrus,
   word comprehension.

### Lesions in frontal lobe may result in:

1  Personality change – apathetic or disinhibited
2  Broca's aphasia (expressive)
3  Abnormal affective reactions
4  Primitive reflexes (e.g. grasp, pout)
5  Perseveration.

### Parietal lobe damage may result in (all the 'A's):

1  Apraxia
2  Acalculia
3  Agraphia
4  Drawing apraxia
5  Constructional apraxia
6  Astereognosis
7  Visual field defects – usually homonymous inferior quadrantanopia.

**Occipital lesions may result in:**

1 Cortical blindness
2 Homonymous hemianopia
3 Visual agnosia (inability to comprehend memory of objects).

**Temporal lobe lesions may result in:**

1 Wernicke's aphasia (receptive)
2 Cortical deafness
3 Memory impairment
4 Impaired musical perception
5 Emotional disturbance – limbic cortex damage
6 Visual field – homonymous superior quadrantanopia.

# The cerebellum

1 Signs of cerebellar pathology:
   (a) Ataxia (wide-based gait)
   (b) Nystagmus
   (c) Dysarthria (scanning speech)
   (d) Dysdiadochokinesia
   (e) Past-pointing
   (f) Intention tremor
2 Causes of cerebellar pathology:
   (a) Alcoholism
   (b) Demyelination (MS)
   (c) Vascular
   (d) Drugs (phenytoin)
   (e) Neoplastic lesions of the posterior fossa
   (f) Congenital syndromes (Friedreich's ataxia)
   (g) Paraneoplastic lesions.

# Functional anatomy of the spinal cord

1 Corticospinal tract:
   (a) Descending motor pathways
   (b) Decussates in the midbrain

2 Dorsal (posterior) columns:
  (a) Ascending sensory pathway
  (b) Joint position sense and vibration sense
  (c) Synapse in the medulla then decussate
3 Spinothalamic tracts:
  (a) Ascending sensory pathway
  (b) Pain and temperature
  (c) Cross immediately or within a few segments.

# Upper motor neurone lesions

1 Lesion above the level of the anterior horn cell
2 Signs:
  (a) Increased tone
  (b) Increased reflexes
  (c) Weakness with little wasting
  (d) Extensor plantar.

# Lower motor neurone lesions

1 Lesion of cell bodies or axons of anterior horn cells
2 Signs:
  (a) Reduced tone
  (b) Absent reflexes
  (c) Fasciculation
  (d) Wasting.

# Dementia

1 An acquired, global impairment of intellect, memory and personality
2 Usually untreatable and progressive
3 Causes of dementia:
  (a) Alzheimer's disease
  (b) Multi-infarct dementia
  (c) Chronic alcoholism
  (d) Pick's disease

    (e)  Huntington's disease
    (f)  Parkinson's disease
    (g)  Lewy-body dementia
    (h)  Creutzfeld–Jakob disease (CJD)
    (i)  AIDS-associated
4 Potentially treatable causes of dementia:
    (a)  $B_{12}$ deficiency
    (b)  Folate deficiency
    (c)  Wilson's disease
    (d)  Hypothyroidism
    (e)  Normal-pressure hydrocephalus.

## Alzheimer's disease

1 Progressive short-term memory loss and cognitive impairment
2 Disorientation and personality changes
3 Classic microscopic appearance of neurofibrillary tangles (tau protein) and senile plaques ($\beta$-amyloid)
4 Loss of cholinergic neurones
5 Affects 5% of over-65s, 20% of over-80s
6 5% are familial (AD)
7 Individuals with Down's syndrome develop Alzheimer's disease early (amyloid precursor protein APP found on chromosome 21).

# Parkinson's disease

1 Degeneration of neurones in substantia nigra (primary or idiopathic)
2 Other causes:
    (a)  Antidopaminergic drugs (neuroleptics)
    (b)  Cerebrovascular disease
    (c)  Postencephalitic
    (d)  Multi-system atrophy
3 Clinical features:
    (a)  Tremor (pill-rolling)
    (b)  Rigidity (cog-wheel, lead-pipe)
    (c)  Bradykinesia
    (d)  Expressionless face
    (e)  Festinant gait (shuffling, lack of arm swing, difficulty starting/stopping/turning)

(f) Dementia (Lewy-body)
4 Treatment:
  (a) L-dopa – dopamine replacement
  (b) Bromocriptine, apomorphine, ropinirole – dopamine agonist
  (c) Selegiline – monoamine-oxidase-B inhibitor
  (d) Benzhexol – anticholinergic
  (e) Pramipexole – catechol-O-methyltransferase inhibitor
  (f) Multidisciplinary team – physiotherapy, speech therapy etc.

# Cerebrovascular disease

1 Transient ischaemic attacks (TIAs):
  (a) Acute focal neurological disturbance that completely recovers within 24 hours
  (b) Embolic
  (c) Symptoms depend on which part of the cerebral circulation is occluded
2 Stroke (cerebrovascular accident, CVA)
  (a) Clinically as for TIA but deficit persists
  (b) Embolic
  (c) Thrombotic
  (d) Haemorrhagic
3 Risk factors (CVA and TIA) (see also risk factors for IHD, in Cardiology):
  (a) Diabetes
  (b) Hypertension
  (c) Smoking
  (d) Previous TIA or CVA
  (e) AF, valvular disease, ischaemic heart disease
  (f) Male sex
  (g) Family history
  (h) Raised haemoglobin
  (i) Oral contraceptive pill
4 Diagnosis:
  (a) Clinical
  (b) CT brain
  (c) MRI of the brain (particularly if cerebellar)
5 Other investigations:
  (a) blood pressure

    (b)  Glucose
    (c)  Cholesterol
    (d)  ESR (temporal arteritis)
    (e)  Carotid Doppler (if carotid territory) to exclude carotid stenosis
    (f)  Echocardiogram to exclude cardiac source of embolus
6  Treatment/secondary prevention:
    (a)  Conservative
    (b)  Aspirin or other antiplatelet drug (if not haemorrhagic)
    (c)  Anticoagulation if AF, mitral stenosis, mural thrombus
    (d)  Treat reversible risk factors
    (e)  Thrombolysis (within 3 hours of onset) in some centres
    (f)  Carotid endarterectomy if >80% stenosis of internal carotid artery
    (g)  Multidisciplinary treatment on Stroke Units (physiotherapy, speech therapy, etc.)
7  Prognosis:
    (a)  Mortality 20–30%
    (b)  25–30% remains significantly disabled
    (c)  Poor outcome:
        (i)   Greater age
        (ii)  Coma at onset
        (iii) Persistent neglect.

## Subarachnoid haemorrhage (SAH)

1  Presents with sudden-onset headache and/or coma
2  5–10% all strokes
3  Causes:
    (a)  Rupture of aneurysm – 80% are of the anterior circulation (mainly anterior communicating artery)
    (b)  Arteriovenous malformation
    (c)  Trauma
    (d)  Cocaine or amphetamine abuse
4  10% of patients with polycystic kidneys have a berry aneurysm
5  Diagnosis:
    (a)  CT scan (but misses 2% of SAH)
    (b)  Lumbar puncture:
        (i)   Xanthochromia (more than 4 hours post-episode)
        (ii)  Red cell count on microscopy
6  Treatment:

(a) Nimodipine – reduces vasospasm
(b) Neurosurgical clipping of the aneurysm
(c) Angiography and embolisation.

# Headache

1 Common causes:
   (a) Tension headaches
   (b) Migraine
   (c) Cluster headaches
   (d) Head injury
   (e) Cervical spondylosis
   (f) Sinusitis
   (g) Drugs (GTN, alcohol)
2 Less common causes:
   (a) Meningitis/encephalitis
   (b) Subarachnoid haemorrhage
   (c) Space-occupying lesion (tumour, abscess, haematoma etc.)
   (d) Temporal arteritis
   (e) $CO_2$ retention
   (f) Glaucoma
   (g) Malignant hypertension
   (h) Benign intracranial hypertension
   (i) Post-lumbar puncture
   (j) Paget's disease.

## Migraine

1 Unilateral, throbbing headache preceded by visual aura
2 Exacerbated by exertion
3 Nausea and vomiting common
4 Photophobia
5 Reversible neurological signs (rare)
6 Vascular in origin – unsure of exact cause
7 Treatment (specific):
   (a) During an attack:
       (i) Sumatriptan
       (ii) Ergotamine
   (b) Prophylaxis:

(i)   Propanolol
(ii)  Pizotifen
(iii) Amitryptiline.

# Neurological infections

## Causes of meningitis

1 Acute bacterial causes:
   (a) Adults:
       (i)   Meningococcus
       (ii)  Pneumococcus
       (iii) *Haemophilus influenzae*
   (b) Neonates:
       (i)  Group B *Streptococcus*
       (ii) *Escherichia* coli
   (c) Rarities (lymphocytic CSF):
       (i)   *Mycobacterium tuberculosis*
       (ii)  *Listeria monocytogenes*
       (iii) Leptospirosis
       (iv)  *Mycoplasma*
       (v)   Syphilis
       (vi)  Lyme disease
2 Chronic bacterial cause: *Mycobacterium tuberculosis*
3 Chronic Fungal causes: cryptococcosis
4 Acute viral causes:
   (a) Mumps
   (b) Enteroviruses (especially polio)
   (c) HSV
   (d) VZV
   (e) HIV.

## Causes of encephalitis

1 Viral causes:
   (a) Herpes simplex (mainly type 1)
   (b) Enteroviruses, e.g. coxsackie
   (c) Arboviruses, e.g. Japanese B encephalitis
   (d) VZV

(e) HIV
(f) Rabies
(g) Measles
2 Other causes:
(a) Toxoplasmosis
(b) African trypanosomiasis.

# Epilepsy

1 Paroxysmal discharge of neurones
2 Diagnosed – more than one seizure in the absence of a cause
3 Prevalence 0.7%, constant at all ages
4 Incidence greatest in the young and the elderly
5 Types of seizure:
(a) Partial:
    (i) Simple – a focal seizure affecting part of one hemisphere with no loss of consciousness
    (ii) Complex – as above but with loss of consciousness
(b) Generalised:
    (i) Grand mal:
        • Tonic-clonic movements with loss of consciousness
        • Often experience tongue biting and urinary incontinence
        • Patient 'postictal'
    (ii) Petit mal: periods of 'absence' – patient may stop talking for a few seconds and appear vacant, then continue as before
6 Diagnosis:
(a) History vital (particularly from onlookers)
(b) Exclude causes of seizure (including CT/MRI, looking for structural lesions)
(c) EEG may show a focus
7 Treatments:
(a) Status epilepticus:
    (i) Intravenous. or rectal diazepam, lorazepam
    (ii) Intravenous phenytoin
(b) Seizure prevention (>80% require only one drug):
    (i) Valproate (first-line)
    (ii) Carbamazepine
    (iii) Phenytoin

NEUROLOGY

     (iv)  Lamotrigine
     (v)  Vigabatrin
     (vi)  Gabapentin
     (vii) Ethosuximide (absence)

8 Driving: patients must be fit-free for one year before driving (HGV – ten years)

9 Epilepsy and pregnancy:

  (a)  Seizure rate predicted by rate prior to pregnancy
  (b)  Drugs all have teratogenic effects
  (c)  Risks of uncontrolled epilepsy are greater than the effects of the drugs
  (d)  Folic acid supplements decrease incidence of malformation.

# Peripheral nerves

## Mononeuropathies

### Carpal tunnel syndrome

1 Lesion of median nerve at the wrist

2 Symptoms:

  (a)  Numbness and dysaesthesia of radial three-and-a-half fingers
  (b)  Weakness of muscles (LOAF):

     (i)  **L**ateral two lumbricals
     (ii)  **O**pponens pollicis
     (iii) **A**bductor pollicis
     (iv) **F**lexor pollicis brevis

3 Associations:

  (a)  Pregnancy
  (b)  Obesity
  (c)  Hypothyroidism
  (d)  Acromegaly
  (e)  Rheumatoid arthritis

4 Treatment:

  (a)  Steroid injection to flexor retinaculum
  (b)  Surgical decompression.

### Ulnar nerve lesions

1 Cause weakness of:

(a) Hypothenar eminence
(b) Abductor digiti minimi
(c) Median two lumbricals
(d) All interossei

2 Numbness and dysaesthesia of ulnar one-and-a-half fingers.

### Radial nerve lesions (Saturday-night palsy)

1 Weakness of extensors of forearm (wrist drop)
2 Loss of sensation over first dorsal interosseus.

### Common peroneal nerve palsy

1 Presents with:
   (a) Foot drop
   (b) Wasting of anterior tibial and peroneal muscles
   (c) Sensory loss on outside of the calf
2 Causes:
   (a) Compression at the neck of the fibula
   (b) Diabetes/vascular
   (c) Leprosy
   (d) Collagen-vascular diseases.

### Causes of wasting of the small muscles of the hand

1 Arthritis
2 Motor neurone disease
3 Syringomyelia
4 Polyneuropathy
5 Brachial plexus injury
6 Other cervical cord pathology.

### Polyneuropathies

Lead to a symmetrical 'glove and stocking' loss of sensation, with distal wasting and weakness. Causes:
   1 Diabetes mellitus
   2 Vitamin $B_{12}$ deficiency
   3 Vitamin $B_1$ deficiency (alcoholics)
   4 Paraneoplastic syndrome
   5 Hereditary sensory and motor neuropathies

NEUROLOGY

    6 HIV
    7 Guillain–Barré syndrome
    8 Sarcoidosis
    9 Leprosy
    10 Vasculitis (RA, PAN, Wegener's granulomatosis)
    11 Drugs:
       (a) Alcohol
       (b) Isoniazid
       (c) Metronidazole
       (d) Amiodarone.

### Guillain–Barré syndrome

1 Acute post-infective polyneuropathy (upper respiratory tract infection, EBV, CMV, *Campylobacter*)
2 Ascending symmetrical progressive muscle weakness leading to paralysis of all four limbs
3 Areflexia
4 Mild sensory symptoms
5 Respiratory muscles affected so artificial ventilation usually required
6 Progresses over a period of less than four weeks
7 Investigation findings:
   (a) Raised CSF proteins
   (b) Normal CSF white cell count
   (c) Slowing of nerve conduction
   (d) Electromyography shows denervation
8 Treatment:
   (a) Intravenous immunoglobulins
   (b) Plasma exchange
   (c) Artificial ventilation.

# Motor neurone disease (MND)

1 Progressive neurodegenerative disease affecting anterior horn cells
2 Purely motor
3 Three patterns of disease:
   (a) Progressive muscular atrophy
   (b) Progressive bulbar palsy
   (c) Primary lateral sclerosis

4 Presentation:
   (a) Limb weakness and wasting
   (b) Muscle fasciculation
   (c) Bulbar palsy
   (d) Respiratory failure (type II)
5 Investigation:
   (a) Diagnosis is clinical
   (b) Electromyography and nerve conduction studies reveal anterior horn cell damage
6 Prognosis poor – life expectancy with bulbar symptoms is two years.

# The cranial nerves

## Visual field loss

**Table 28**

| Lesions affecting one eye (indicates ocular, retinal or optic nerve pathology) | |
| --- | --- |
| Complete visual loss | Ipsilateral optic nerve transection |
| Central scotoma (hole in vision) | Optic nerve disease e.g. neuritis |
| Constricted field | Chronic papilloedema, chronic glaucoma |

| Lesions affecting both eyes (indicates lesion at or behind the optic chiasm) | |
| --- | --- |
| Bitemporal hemianopia | Chiasmal lesion |
| | Pituitary adenoma |
| | Crainopharyngioma |
| | Intracranial aneurysm |
| | Meningioma |
| Homonymous quadrantanopia | Superior – temporal lobe lesion |
| | Inferior – parietal lobe lesion |
| Homonymous hemianopia | Incongruous – lesion of the optic tract |
| | Congruous – lesion of lateral geniculate body |
| | Macular sparing – lesion of optic cortex |

## The pupil

1 Pupilloconstrictor (parasympathetic) fibres
2 Pupillodilator (sympathetic) fibres.

### Causes of a small pupil (miosis)

1 Horner's syndrome
2 Argyll Robertson pupil – do not react to light but normal accommodation reaction
3 Senile miosis
4 Drugs, e.g. opiates, pilocarpine.

### Causes of a large pupil (mydriasis)

1 Adie's pupil – idiopathic, reacts poorly to light. Decreased tendon reflexes (Holmes–Adie pupil)
2 Third nerve palsy
3 Drugs – amphetamines, antidepressants, tropicamide, atropine
4 Trauma.

### Horner's syndrome

1 Features:
   (a) Miosis
   (b) Enophthalmos
   (c) Ptosis
   (d) Anhidrosis
2 Causes (lesions may occur throughout the course of the sympathetic trunk):
   (a) Lesions of brainstem or spinal cord:
      (i) Vascular
      (ii) Trauma
      (iii) Neoplastic
      (iv) Demyelination
      (v) Syringomyelia
   (b) Preganglonic lesion:
      (i) Chest – apical carcinoma, cervical rib, mediastinal mass
      (ii) Cervical – lymphadenopathy, trauma, thyroid neoplasm, neck surgery
   (c) Postganglionic lesion:
      (i) Internal carotid artery dissection
      (ii) Cavernous sinus lesion
      (iii) Orbital apex disease.

## Third nerve palsy

1 Features:
  (a) Ptosis
  (b) Inability to move the eye superiorly, inferiorly, medially
  (c) Eye: down and out
  (d) Pupil fixed and dilated
2 Causes:
  (a) Vascular/diabetes/demyelination/trauma
  (b) Posterior communicating artery aneurysm
  (c) Cavernous sinus thrombosis
  (d) Orbital tumour
  (e) Thyroid eye disease
  (f) Trauma.

## Fourth nerve palsy (superior oblique)

1 Fourth nerve exits dorsal aspect of brainstem (only one to do so)
2 Diplopia when descending stairs or reading
3 Causes:
  (a) Vascular/diabetes/demyelination/trauma
  (b) Congenital
  (c) Cavernous sinus syndrome
  (d) Orbital apex syndrome.

## Sixth nerve palsy (lateral rectus)

1 Diplopia on lateral gaze (towards affected side)
2 Affected eye deviates medially
3 Causes:
  (a) Raised intracranial pressure (false localising sign).
  (b) Vascular/diabetes/demyelination/trauma
  (c) Cavernous sinus
  (d) Orbital apex disease.

## The facial nerve

1 Functions:
  (a) Motor nerves to muscles of facial expression
  (b) Chorda tympani to anterior two-thirds of tongue
  (c) Parasympathetic fibres to parotid, submandibular and sublingual

glands
   (d)  Supplies stapedius muscle in the ear
2  Causes of facial nerve palsy:
   (a)  Vascular/diabetes/demyelination/trauma
   (b)  Bell's palsy
   (c)  Ramsay Hunt syndrome – herpes zoster infection
   (d)  Guillain–Barré syndrome
   (e)  Acoustic neuroma
   (f)  Brainstem tumour.

# Movement disorders

### Causes of chorea

1  Huntington's disease
2  Sydenham's chorea (rheumatic)
3  Drugs (neuroleptics, phenytoin)
4  SLE
5  Thyrotoxicosis
6  Pregnancy (chorea gravidarum)
7  Wilson's disease
8  Cerebellar degeneration.

### Huntington's disease

1  Autosomal dominant – chromosome 4
2  Presents between the ages of 35 and 50 with:
   (a)  Chorea
   (b)  Cognitive decline
3  Positive family history (implications as patient has usually had children by then).

# Muscular disorders

### Duchenne muscular dystrophy

1  X-linked; 1 in 3500 male births
2  Absence of dystrophin protein in muscle
3  Delay in motor milestones

4  Proximal muscles mostly affected
5  Pseudohypertrophy of calf muscles
6  Ability to walk lost at around 12 years old
7  Death by respiratory/cardiac failure in the 20s or early 30s.


## Myotonic dystrophy

1  Myotonic facies
2  Myotonia (unable to relax muscles following contraction)
3  Progressive muscular weakness and wasting, starting distally
4  Frontal balding
5  Bilateral ptosis
6  Cataracts
7  Diabetes
8  Respiratory muscle weakness (type II respiratory failure)
9  Mental retardation (in severe cases)
10  Testicular/ovarian atrophy.


## Myasthenia gravis

1  Antibodies to acetylcholine receptors on postsynaptic membrane of neuromuscular junction
2  Leads to increased muscle fatiguability
3  70–80% have pathological changes in the thymus gland (20% thymoma)
4  Symptoms and signs:
   (a)  Ptosis
   (b)  Ophthalmoplegia
   (c)  Dysarthria
   (d)  Fatiguable weakness of striated muscle
   (e)  Respiratory muscle involvement is life-threatening
5  Investigations:
   (a)  Acetylcholine receptor antibodies (in around 90%)
   (b)  Electromyography (EMG) – decreasing muscle action potential with repetitive motor nerve stimulation
   (c)  Tensilon test – intravenous edrophonium assesses immediate- and short-acting effect of anticholinesterases
   (d)  CT thorax – ? associated thymoma
6  Treatment:
   (a)  Pyridostigmine (cholinesterase inhibitor), lifelong treatment

(b) Thymectomy
(c) Immunosuppression.

# Multiple sclerosis (MS)

1 Demyelinating disease
2 Cell-mediated autoimmune disease associated with immune activity against myelin
3 Four subtypes:
    (a) Relapsing/remitting disease: 80–85% of patients
    (b) Primary progressive disease: 10–15%, deterioration from onset
    (c) Secondary progressive disease: 30–50% of patients with relapsing/remitting form
    (d) Progressive relapsing disease: superimposed relapses:
4 Symptoms:
    (a) Weakness (40%)
    (b) Optic neuritis (22%)
    (c) Paraesthesiae (21%)
    (d) Diplopia (12%)
    (e) Disturbance of micturition (5%)
    (f) Vertigo (5%)
5 Diagnosis:
    (a) Two or more CNS demyelinating lesions (in time and place)
    (b) Diagnosis not possible at time of first neurological event
6 Investigations:
    (a) MRI scan
    (b) Delayed visual-evoked response potentials
    (c) Oligoclonal bands in CSF (non-specific)
7 Management:
    (a) Intravenous methylprednisolone for acute attacks
    (b) Interferon-$\beta$: reduces frequency and severity of relapses
8 Prognosis:
    (a) Disabling paraparesis in 33%
    (b) 10% remain minimally disabled ten years after onset ('benign' MS).

# Cerebrospinal fluid (CSF)

## Causes of raised CSF pressure

1 Space-occupying lesions or acute brain swelling
2 TB meningitis
3 High venous pressure, e.g. dural sinus thrombosis
4 Benign intracranial hypertension
5 Hydrocephalus.

## Increased CSF protein concentration

1 Markedly raised (approximately 2–6 g/l):
  (a) Guillain–Barré syndrome
  (b) Spinal block (secondary to tumour)
  (c) TB meningitis
  (d) Fungal meningitis
2 Raised:
  (a) Bacterial meningitis
  (b) Viral encephalitis
  (c) Cerebral abscess
  (d) Multiple sclerosis
  (e) Cerebral tumours (primary and metastases)
  (f) Cerebral infarction
  (g) Subdural haematoma.

## White cells in CSF

1 Polymorphs: bacterial meningitis
2 Lymphocytes:
  (a) Viral encephalitis/meningitis
  (b) Partially treated bacterial meningitis
  (c) TB.

## Reduced or absent CSF glucose

1 Bacterial meningitis
2 TB meningitis
3 Malignant meningitis, i.e. atypical – fungal meningitis, mumps
4 Herpes simplex encephalitis
5 Subarachnoid haemorrhage.

**Table 29**

|  | Normal CSF | Acute bacterial meningitis | Acute viral meningitis | Mycobacterium tuberculosis infection | Multiple sclerosis |
|---|---|---|---|---|---|
| Appearance | Crystal Clear, colourless | Turbid/purulent | Clear/turbid | Turbid/viscous | Normal |
| Glucose | Two-thirds to one-half of blood glucose | Low | Normal or high | Low | Normal |
| Protein | 0.2–0.4 g/l | Very high | High | Very high | High |
| Mononuclear cells | $5/mm^3$ | $< 50/mm^3$ | $10–100/mm^3$ | $100–300/mm^3$ | $5–60/mm^3$ |
| Polymorphs | Nil | $200–3000/mm^3$ | Nil (early) | $0–200/mm^3$ |  |
| Microbiology | Nil | Gram stain and blood culture etc. | Throat swab and serology etc. | AAFB on ZN staining | IgG >15% of normal Oligoclonal band-positive |
| Pressure | 60–150 mm of $H_2O$ with patient lying down | Normal or raised | Normal or raised | Normal or raised | Normal or raised |

### CSF findings in health and disease

[see Table 29, overleaf]

# Alcohol and the CNS

### Acute alcohol withdrawal (delirium tremens)

1 Tremor
2 Visual hallucinations
3 Acute confusion
4 Insomnia
5 Agitation
6 Pyrexia
7 Onset after 72 hours without alcohol
8 Electrolyte deficiencies often seen (potassium, magnesium)
9 Mortality 5%.

### Wernicke's encephalopathy

1 Due to acute thiamine deficiency
2 Features are:
   (a) Gross confusion
   (b) Ataxia
   (c) Nystagmus
   (d) Abducens and conjugate gaze palsies
3 Microvascular lesions in third and fourth ventricles, peri-aqueductal grey matter, mamillary bodies, brainstem and cerebellum
4 Treat with intravenous thiamine
5 80% develop Korsakoff's syndrome (irreversible, leads to amnesia, lack of insight and confabulation).

# Causes of acute confusional state (delirium)

1 Usually reversible
2 Intracranial:
   (a) Head injury

   (b)  CNS infection (encephalitis, meningitis)
   (c)  Epilepsy
   (d)  Space-occupying lesion
   (e)  Intracranial bleed (subarachnoid, intracerebral, subdural)
   (f)  Cerebrovascular disease
3  Extracranial:
   (a)  Infection (urinary tract, chest)
   (b)  Toxic (alcohol, drugs – prescribed or illicit)
   (c)  Endocrine (thyroid, diabetes, adrenal, especially Cushing's)
   (d)  Electrolyte disorder (sodium, calcium)
   (e)  Metabolic (hypoglycaemia, uraemia, hepatic encephalopathy)
   (f)  Systemic (SLE).

# Ophthalmology

## Eye signs in medical disorders

**Table 30**

| Sign | Disorder |
| --- | --- |
| Lisch nodules | Neurofibromatosis |
| Brushfield spots | Down's syndrome |
| Kayser–Fleischer rings | Wilson's disease |
| Bitot's spots | Vitamin A deficiency |
| Corneal arcus | Hypercholesterolaemia |
| | Old age |
| Blue sclera | Osteogenesis imperfecta |
| | Pseudoxanthoma elasticum |
| | Ehlers–Danlos syndrome |
| | Marfan's syndrome |
| | Hyperthyroidism |
| Corneal calcification | Sarcoidosis |
| | Hyperparathyroidism |
| | Chronic renal failure |
| | Vitamin D abuse |

## Diabetic eye disease

The most common cause of blindness in patients aged 30–60.
1 Background retinopathy:
  (a) Visual acuity unaffected
  (b) Microaneurysms
  (c) Haemorrhages
  (d) Hard exudates
2 Preproliferative retinopathy:
  (a) Cotton-wool spots

187

    (b)  Dilatation and beading of retinal veins
    (c)  Intraretinal microvascular abnormalities
3  Proliferative retinopathy (more common in type 1 diabetics):
    (a)  Neovascularisation
    (b)  Treated cases will have panretinal laser burns
4  Advanced diabetic eye disease:
    (a)  Vitreous haemorrhage
    (b)  Tractional retinal detachment
    (c)  Rubeotic glaucoma
5  Maculopathy (more common in type 2 diabetics):
    (a)  Oedema and exudates
    (b)  Macular stars (multiple exudates)
    (c)  Loss of central vision (peripheral vision spared)
6  Treatment:
    (a)  Good diabetic control
    (b)  Treat hypertension
    (c)  Stop smoking
    (d)  Treat hypercholesterolaemia
    (e)  Regular fundal examination
    (f)  Focal retinal photocoagulation
    (g)  Panretinal photocoagulation.

# Hypertensive retinopathy

*Grade 1*: silver wiring of retinal arteries
*Grade 2*:
1  Arteriovenous nipping
2  Focal arteriolar attenuation
*Grade 3*:
3  Haemorrhages
4  Hard exudates
5  Cotton-wool spots
*Grade 4*: papilloedema.

# Causes of papilloedema

1  Raised intracranial pressure:
    (a)  Space-occupying lesion (tumour, haematoma, abscess)

(b) Meningitis/encephalitis
(c) Subarachnoid haemorrhage
(d) Cerebral oedema
2 Hypertensive retinopathy
3 Benign intracranial hypertension
4 Metabolic causes:
(a) $CO_2$ retention
(b) Vitamin A intoxication
(c) Lead poisoning
5 Central retinal vein thrombosis.

# Causes of optic atrophy

1 Congenital (Leber's optic atrophy, Friedreich's ataxia)
2 Multiple sclerosis
3 Compression of the optic nerve (tumour, aneurysm)
4 Glaucoma
5 Chronic papilloedema
6 Ischaemia (retinal artery occlusion, temporal arteritis)
7 Nutritional deficiency
8 Toxic (methanol)
9 Retinitis pigmentosa
10 Drugs (ethambutol).

# Optic neuritis

1 Inflammation of the optic nerve
2 Unilateral reduction of acuity over hours to days
3 Colours (particularly red) appear less intense
4 Optic disc swollen
5 Recovery over 2–6 weeks
6 45–80% develop MS over the next 15 years
7 Treat with high-dose methylprednisolone for three days.

# Causes of choroidoretinitis

1 CMV

2  Toxoplasmosis
3  Toxocariasis
4  AIDS
5  Sarcoidosis
6  TB.

# Causes of cataracts

1  Congenital:
   (a)  Autosomal dominant
   (b)  Maternal infection (rubella, CMV, toxoplasmosis)
   (c)  Down's syndrome
2  Senile
3  UV light
4  Drugs (steroids)
5  Ocular disease (uveitis, high myopia)
6  Metabolic (diabetes, Cushing's syndrome)
7  Myotonic dystrophy.

# Causes of uveitis

1  Idiopathic
2  Ankylosing spondylitis
3  Reiter's syndrome
4  Psoriatic disease
5  Inflammatory bowel disease
6  Sarcoidosis
7  Juvenile chronic arthritis.
8  Trauma
9  Infections:
   (a)  TB
   (b)  HSV
   (c)  Toxoplasmosis
   (d)  Toxocariasis.

# Causes of ptosis

1 Unilateral:
  (a) Congenital
  (b) Idiopathic
  (c) Third nerve palsy
  (d) Horner's syndrome
  (e) Myasthenia gravis
  (f) Lid tumour
2 Bilateral:
  (a) Myasthenia gravis
  (b) Dystrophica myotonica
  (c) Ocular myopathy
  (d) Bilateral Horner's (syringomyelia).

# Respiratory Medicine

## Respiratory function tests

### Lung volumes and spirometry

1 Total lung capacity (TLC):
   (a) 6–7 litres in the normal adult
   (b) Measured by body plethysmography or helium dilution technique
2 Tidal volume (TV):
   (a) Volume of normal resting breath
   (b) Approximately 500 ml in the normal adult
3 Vital capacity (VC):
   (a) End of forced inspiration to end of forced expiration
   (b) 75% of TLC
   (c) Decreases with age
   (d) Depends on height, age, sex and ethnic origin
4 Forced vital capacity (FVC):
   (a) Volume of maximal forceful expiration after maximal inspiration
   (b) Reduced in restrictive disorders
   (c) May be normal or increased in obstructive disorders
5 Forced expiratory volume$_1$ (FEV$_1$):
   (a) Volume expired in one second of maximal expiration after maximal
       inspiration
   (b) Normal is 75–80% of FVC
   (c) Variables are same as for VC
   (d) Reduced in obstructive airways disease; marker of severity
6 Peak expiratory flow rate (PEFR):
   (a) Flow rate of first 0.01 second of maximal expiration

(b)  Variables as for VC

(c)  Only measures calibre of medium and large airways.

Pulmonary blood flow approximately 5000 ml/minute.
Alveolar ventilation approximately 5250 ml/minute.

## Blood gases

### *Oxygenation of haemoglobin*

1  Haemoglobin changes from ferric to ferrous form
2  Fetal haemoglobin (Hb F) has a greater affinity for oxygen than Hb A
3  Partial pressure of oxygen and saturation ($Sao_2$) follow oxygen dissociation curve
4  Increased affinity for oxygen represents shift of the curve to RIGHT.

### *Causes of increased oxygen affinity*

1  ↑ temperature
2  ↑ $H^+$, i.e. ↓ pH
3  ↑ $Paco_2$
4  ↑ 2,3 diphosphoglycerate (adaptation to altitude, chronic anaemia).

All these changes occur in working muscle.

## Gas transfer factor

1  Measure of gas diffusion across alveolar membrane into capillaries
2  Depends on blood volume, blood flow, surface area of membrane and distribution of ventilation
3  Measured by diffusion of carbon monoxide ($TLco$)
4  $Kco$ is the above, corrected for lung volume.

### *Causes of decreased transfer factor*

1  Chronic obstructive pulmonary disease (COPD)
2  Interstitial lung disease
3  Pulmonary embolus
4  Pneumonia
5  Pulmonary oedema
6  Pneumonectomy.

*Causes of increased transfer factor*

1 Pulmonary haemorrhage
2 Polycythaemia
3 Left–right shunt.

# Respiratory failure

### Type I

Hypoxaemia ($Po_2 < 8$ kPa / 60 mmHg) with normal $Pco_2$

1 Causes:
   (a) Early stages of severe asthma
   (b) Emphysema
   (c) Pneumonia
   (d) Pulmonary embolus
   (e) Pulmonary oedema
   (f) Interstitial lung disease
   (g) Acute respiratory distress syndrome
2 Treatment – increasing inspired $Fio_2$.

### Type II

Hypoxaemia with $CO_2$ retention ($Pco_2 > 6.7$ kPa / 50 mmHg).

1 Causes:
   (a) COPD
   (b) Late stages of severe asthma
   (c) Neurological disorders (Guillaine–Barré, MND, MS)
   (d) Muscular disease (myasthenia gravis, muscular dystrophy)
   (e) Chest wall disease (kyphoscoliosis, ankylosing spondylitis, surgery)
   (f) Drugs (opioids)
2 Treatment:
   (a) Usually require mechanical ventilatory support
   (b) Respiratory stimulants (doxepram) of limited use.

# Asthma

## Chronic asthma

1 Incidence 20% in children, 15% in adults
2 Chronic inflammatory disorder with variable airflow obstruction
3 Combination of genetic predisposition and environmental atopy
4 Pulmonary function tests:
  (a)  $>25\%$ variation in PEFR
  (b)  $\downarrow$ FEV$_1$
  (c)  $\downarrow$ FEV$_1$/FVC ratio
  (d)  PEFR and FEV$_1$ $\uparrow$ post-bronchodilator
  (e)  $\uparrow$ lung volume
5 Acute attack provoked by:
  (a)  Exposure to allergen (pollen, house-dust mite, cat and dog dander)
  (b)  Exercise
  (c)  Drugs (NSAIDs and aspirin, beta-blockers)
  (d)  Infection
  (e)  Oesophageal reflux
  (f)  Smoke
  (g)  Non-compliance with medication
6 Treatment of chronic asthma (escalation of therapy) – BTS guidelines:
  (a)  Short-acting beta-agonists, e.g. salbutamol, as required
  (b)  Add low-dose steroid inhaler, e.g. beclomethasone 100–400 μg twice daily OR leukotriene antagonists, e.g. montelukast
  (c)  High-dose steroid inhaler, e.g. beclomethasone 500–1000 μg OR low-dose steroid inhaler and long-acting beta-agonist, e.g. salmeterol twice daily
  (d)  Add $>1$ of long-acting beta-agonists, oral theophylline, inhaled ipratropium, regular high-dose inhaled bronchodilators (nebulisers)
  (e)  Intermittant or maintenance oral steroids.

## Acute asthma

Causes around 1500 deaths per year in the UK.
1 Markers of severe acute asthma:
  (a)  Difficulty speaking
  (b)  Tachycardia $>$ 110 bpm

 (c) Pulsus paradoxus
 (d) Respiratory rate $> 30$/minute
 (e) PFFR $< 33\%$ of best/predicted
 (f) Silent chest
 (g) Hypoxia
 (h) Normal or raised $P_{CO_2}$
2 Management:
 (a) High-flow $O_2$
 (b) Nebulised bronchodilators
 (c) Steroids
 (d) Intravenous aminophylline or salbutamol
 (e) Ventilation.

## Causes of occupational asthma

1 Isocyanates (paint, plastics, insulation)
2 Flour and grain dusts
3 Soldering flux (colophony fumes)
4 Epoxy resins
5 Proteolytic enzymes (detergents manufacture).

# Chronic obstructive pulmonary disease (COPD)

1 Chronic progressive disorder characterised by fixed airflow obstruction that does not change markedly over several months
2 Biggest aetiological factor is smoking
3 Patients have varying degrees of chronic bronchitis and emphysema
4 Chronic bronchitis is a clinical diagnosis of productive cough lasting for three months in two consecutive years
5 Emphysema is an pathological diagnosis with destruction of the acinus (but features can be seen on CT)
6 Alpha-1-antitrypsin deficiency also a cause
7 Marked morbidity/mortality
8 Clinical features:
 (a) Cough (usually productive)
 (b) Breathlessness

    (c) Wheeze

    (d) Recurrent exacerbations

**Table 31**

| Pink puffer | Blue bloater |
|---|---|
| Hyperventilation | Hypoventilation |
| ↓ $PaCO_2$ (type I resp failure) | ↑ $PaCO_2$ (type II resp failure) |
| Breathless but not cyanosed | Cyanosed but not breathless<br>Cor pulmonale |

9  $FEV_1$/FVC ratio <75%; $FEV_1$ <80% of predicted

10  Treatment (BTS guidelines):

    (a) Acute – as for asthma – but oxygen therapy must be controlled as some patients have type II respiratory failure

    (b) Chronic:

        (i)   Stopping smoking (only measure that will slow progression)

        (ii)  Influenza vaccine

        (iii) Mild disease ($FEV_1$ 60–80%) – short-acting beta-agonist or ipratropium as required

        (iv) Moderate disease ($FEV_1$ 40–59%):

          • Regular short-acting beta-agonist or ipratropium

          • Consider corticosteroid trial, if reversibility (>15 % improvement in $FEV_1$) then give steroid inhaler

        (v)  Severe disease ($FEV_1$ <40%):

          • Nebuliser trial

          • Consider long-term oxygen therapy if: non-smoker, $PaO_2$ <7.3 kPa, $FEV_1$ < 1.5 litres on maximal treatment OR $PaO_2$ 7.3–8.0 kPa with evidence of pulmonary hypertension

11  Complications:

    (a) Respiratory failure

    (b) Recurrent 'exacerbations'

    (c) Cor pulmonale

    (d) Polycythaemia

    (e) Pneumothorax

    (f) Lung cancer (smoking)

    (g) Osteoporosis (steroids).

### Alpha-1-antitrypsin deficiency

1 Autosomal codominant
2 Most severe with ZZ deficiency
3 Presents in third to fourth decades
4 Marked panlobular emphysema in basal lung areas
5 Worse in smokers
6 Associated with liver cirrhosis.

# Bronchiectasis

Irreversible dilatation of small airways. Obstructive spirometry due to plugging by secretions.

### Causes

1 Congenital:
  (a) Cystic fibrosis
  (b) Selective IgA deficiency
  (c) Kartagener's syndrome (ciliary dyskinesis associated with infertility, dextrocardia and situs inversus)
  (d) Primary immotile cilia syndrome
  (e) X-linked hypogammaglobulinaemia
2 Acquired:
  (a) Childhood pneumonia, pertussis, measles
  (b) Post-TB
  (c) Allergic bronchopulmonary aspergillosis (ABPA)
  (d) Distal to obstructed bronchus (foreign body, tumour)
  (e) Associated with pulmonary fibrosis and sarcoid
  (f) Idiopathic.

### Features

1 Chronic production of purulent sputum
2 Exertional breathlessness
3 Clubbing
4 Early/mid-inspiratory crepitations
5 CXR shows thickened bronchial walls and ring shadows
6 Obstructive or restrictive spirometry
7 High-resolution CT is usually diagnostic.

# Cystic fibrosis

1   Autosomal recessive inheritance
2   1 in 25 adults are carriers
3   Incidence 1 in 2000 live births
4   Gene on long arm of chromosome 7 codes for cystic fibrosis transmembrane regulator protein (CFTR)
5   Defect of chloride and water transport across the epithelial cell membrane
6   Diagnosis by sweat test: sodium and chloride concentrations > 60 mmol/l
7   Life expectancy now reaching the forties
8   Respiratory features:
   (a)   Obstruction of small airways with thick mucus due to decreased chloride secretion and increased sodium resorption
   (b)   Colonisation with *Staphylococcus aureus, Haemophilus influenzae* and *Pseudomonas aeruginosa*
   (c)   *Burkholderia cepacia* increasingly important, highly transmissible
   (d)   Chronic infection and inflammation with bronchiectasis
   (e)   Respiratory failure in late stages
   (f)   Treat with antibiotics, acutely and prophylactically, oral ± nebulised
   (g)   Transplantation
9   Gastrointestinal features:
   (a)   Pancreatic insufficiency in 80% (steatorrhoea, vitamin deficiency): oral pancreatic supplements given
   (b)   Meconium ileus in infancy, small bowel obstruction in adults
   (c)   Chronic liver disease seen due to biliary tree obstruction ( < 5%)
   (d)   Gallstones
   (e)   Pancreatitis
10  Other features:
   (a)   Diabetes ( > 30% of patients in late teens)
   (b)   Nasal polyps (30%)
   (c)   Pneumothorax (5%)
   (d)   Infertility (almost all men)
   (e)   Osteoporosis.

# Pulmonary fibrosis

## Causes

**Table 32**

| Upper lobe fibrosis | Sarcoidosis |
| --- | --- |
| | TB |
| | Pneumoconiosis |
| | Silicosis |
| | Ankylosing spondylitis |
| | ABPA |
| Lower lobe fibrosis | Bronchiectasis |
| | Asbestosis |
| | CFA |
| | RA |
| | Drugs |
| | Systemic sclerosis |
| | Radiation |

### *Drugs that cause pulmonary fibrosis*

1 Amiodarone
2 Methotrexate
3 Nitrofurantoin
4 Bleomycin.

### Idiopathic pulmonary fibrosis (cryptogenic fibrosing alveolitis or CFA)

1 Chronic inflammatory condition of alveoli leading to lung fibrosis
2 Commoner in men
3 Features: dry cough, breathlessness, clubbing, cyanosis, fine late-inspiratory crepitations
4 Restrictive spirometry, bibasal interstitial shadowing on CXR, type I respiratory failure
5 Characteristic features on CT for diagnosis.

# Extrinsic allergic alveolitis

IgG-mediated type III and IV hypersensitivity reaction to inhaled particles.

Causes pneumonitis.

## Causes

1 Farmer's lung: thermophilic actinomyces (*Micropolyspora faeni* and *Thermoactinomyces vulgaris*) in mouldy hay
2 Bird fancier's lung: seen in keepers of pigeons and budgerigars. Due to keratin in faeces and feather bloom
3 Malt worker's lung: *Aspergillus clavatus*
4 Mushroom worker's lung: thermophilic actinomyces.

## Features

1 Fever, cough and breathlessness 4–9 hours after exposure. No wheeze. Settles in 48 hours
2 CXR may be normal; may have nodular shadows and hazy infiltrate
3 Chronic disease causes irreversible fibrosis and restrictive spirometry
4 Serum precipitins helpful in diagnosis
5 No eosinophilia
6 Bronchoalveolar lavage or transbronchial biopsy may help in diagnosis
7 Treatment is avoidance of precipitant, and steroids in acute illness (though no improvement in outcome in chronic disease).

# Occupational lung disease

### Coal-worker's pneumoconiosis (CWP)

1 Occurs 10–20 years after exposure
2 Small particles retained in alveoli and small bronchioles
3 Show as small rounded opacities in lung fields
4 Background CWP may go on to progressive massive fibrosis (PMF)
5 Large opacities > 10 mm in PMS. Usually upper lobe. May cavitate
6 Mixed obstructive/restrictive pattern
7 Compensatable (only if there are CXR changes)
8 Caplan's syndrome – multiple lung nodules in a patient with rheumatoid arthritis and CWP. Usually peripheral.

## Silicosis

1 Inhaled silicon dioxide in rock-face miners, quarry workers, engineers and sandblasters
2 Subacute phase occurs within a few months of exposure – breathlessness and dry cough
3 Progresses to upper lobe nodule formation
4 Late stages – restrictive lung disease
5 Previously showed a marked increase in TB
6 Only treatment is transplant
7 Compensatable.

## Diseases caused by exposure to asbestos

1 Pleural plaques and thickening:
   (a) Occurs 20 years or more after exposure
   (b) Plaques on parietal pleura
   (c) Usually asymptomatic
   (d) May progress to diffuse confluent thickening, causing exertional breathlessness
   (e) Restrictive spirometry, Kco normal
2 Asbestosis:
   (a) Occurs 20 years or more after exposure
   (b) Lower lobe fibrosis
   (c) Dry cough, exertional breathlessness, lower-zone crepitations and clubbing
   (d) CXR shows irregular shadowing, with ring and honeycomb patterns in later disease
   (e) Restrictive spirometry and low Kco
   (f) Associated with increased incidence of lung cancer
   (g) Compensatable
3 Mesothelioma:
   (a) 85% of cases due to asbestos
   (b) See below in section on lung cancer.

# Granulomatous lung disease

## Sarcoidosis

1 Multisystem disease

2  Cause unknown
3  Mainly affects young adults
4  Three times more common in Blacks
5  Characteristic lesion is a non-caseating granuloma.

### Symptoms

1  There may be no respiratory symptoms
2  Dry cough, fever, breathlessness, weight loss
3  Examination often shows nothing significant, occasional clubbing
4  Bilateral hilar lymphadenopathy and erythema nodosum – almost diagnostic
5  May progress to irreversible fibrosis – upper and mid-zones usually affected
6  May rarely see upper airway involvement with obstruction and discharge.

### Chest X-ray classification

Stage 0 – Normal CXR
Stage 1 – Bilateral hilar lymphadenopathy (BHL)
Stage 2 – BHL and pulmonary infiltrates
Stage 3 – Diffuse infiltration

### Diagnosis

1  Transbronchial biopsy diagnostic in 85% of stage 1 cases
2  Raised calcium and ACE levels.

### Extrapulmonary manifestations

1  Liver (40–70%) – subclinical granuloma infiltration
2  Cardiac (30–70%) – cardiac muscle problems, arrhythmias
3  Skin (25%) – erythema nodosum, nodules, lupus pernio
4  Eyes (25%) – anterior uveitis
5  Splenomegaly (25%)
6  Neurological (5%) – meningitis, space-occupying lesions, cranial nerve palsy; may affect posterior pituitary
7  Bone – cysts (small bones of hands and feet), arthritis (Löfgrens syndrome – triad of BHL, polyarthritis and erythema nodosum).

### Treatment

1  May not need any treatment
2  Steroids
3  Azathioprine, methotrexate.

### Prognosis

Stage 1 – 80% spontaneous remission
Stage 2 – 30% spontaneous remission.

# Lung cancer

The commonest cancer in the West.

## Causes

1  Smoking (95%)
2  Industrial (asbestos, arsenic, benzoyl chloride, aluminium salts)
3  Atmospheric (pollution, passive smoking).

## Cell types

1  Squamous (52%): arise in the central airway
2  Small cell (21%): central airway, rapidly growing and early metastasis
3  Adenocarcinoma (11%): may be peripheral
4  Large cell (10%)
5  Bronchiolar-alveolar cell (6%).

## Complications

1  Physical\metastatic:
    (a)  Pleural effusion
    (b)  Dysphagia
    (c)  Superior vena cava obstruction
    (d)  Recurrent laryngeal nerve palsy → hoarseness
    (e)  Phrenic nerve palsy → raised hemidiaphragm
    (f)  Pericarditis and effusion
    (g)  Spontaneous pneumothorax
2  Non-metastatic:

    (a)  SIADH (small cell)
    (b)  Ectopic ACTH (small cell)
    (c)  Hypercalcaemia (metastases, squamous cell mediated by PTHrP)
    (d)  Gynaecomastia (large cell)
    (e)  Clubbing (commonest in non-small cell)
    (f)  Eaton–Lambert syndrome (small cell): proximal myopathy and reduced tendon reflexes
    (g)  Hypertrophic pulmonary osteoarthropathy (squamous cell): arthritis, clubbing and periostitis. Commonly affects long bones
3 Treatment:
    (a)  Surgery for non-small cell. Only 20% are operable. Five-year survival post-surgery only 25%
    (b)  Palliative/radical radiotherapy
    (c)  Chemotherapy, particularly for small cell tumours
4 Prognosis:
    (a)  Median survival for small-cell tumours is 14 months in limited disease, 10 months in extensive disease
    (b)  Five-year survival for non-small-cell tumours is 10% with treatment.

## Mesothelioma

(a)  There are 1000 cases per year in the UK
(b)  Commonest in men
(c)  85% due to asbestos exposure
(d)  Blue (crocidolite) > brown (amosite) > white (crysotile)
(e)  Presents 20 – 50 years after exposure
(f)  No cure
(g)  Median survival 16 months.

# Pneumonia

## Community-acquired pneumonia

1 Incidence is 3 per 1000 per year
2 Causal organisms:
    (a)  *Streptococcus pneumoniae* (60–75%)
    (b)  Atypical organisms (5–18%):
        (i)  *Mycoplasma pneumoniae*

   (ii)  *Legionella*
   (iii) *Chlamydia psittaci* and *Chlamydia pneumoniae*
(c)  *Haemophilus influenzae* (5%)
(d)  *Staphylococcus aureus*
(e)  *Moraxella catarrhalis*
(f)  Viruses (influenza, parainfluenza, varicella, RSV).

## *Mycoplasma* pneumonia

1 Affects young adults
2 Epidemics every 3–4 years
3 Long prodromal phase
4 May be associated with cold agglutinins.

## *Legionella* pneumonia

1 Contaminated air-conditioning, showers, water cooling systems
2 There is often underlying lung disease
3 WCC may be normal, with lymphopenia
4 SIADH and low sodium
5 Abnormal LFTs in 50%
6 Neurological signs and symptoms common.

## *Staphylococcus* pneumonia

1 May complicate influenza
2 Common in intravenous drug absusers
3 Associated with lung abscess and empyema.

## Markers of severity in pneumonia (BTS guidelines) – severe if > 2 of:

1 Diastolic BP < 60 mmHg
2 Serum urea > 7 mmol/l
3 Repiratory rate > 30/minute.

## Hospital-acquired pneumonia

Organisms:
1 *S. aureus*
2 Gram-negative organisms (*Klebsiella*, *Proteus*, *E. coli*, *Pseudomonas*)

3 Anaerobes.

## Treatment of pneumonia

1 Be guided by microbiology
2 If *Streptococcus pneumoniae* – amoxicillin
3 If an atypical organism or penicillin-allergic – clarithromycin
4 If hospital-acquired use third-generation cephalosporin to cover Gram negatives
5 If *S. aureus* – flucloxicillin (teicoplanin or vancomycin if MRSA).

# Tuberculosis

Incidence is increasing.

## At-risk groups

1 Immigrants from endemic areas
2 Alcoholics
3 HIV-positive
4 Homeless
5 Low income.

## Primary TB

1 May be entirely asymptomatic
2 Infection in a person with no immunity
3 Ghon focus develops in the lung
4 Bacilli are transported through lymphatics
5 Infection is then arrested
6 Tuberculin tests become positive after this
7 May cause mild cough, wheeze and erythema nodosum.

## Post-primary TB

Reactivation of disseminated dormant organisms.

## Miliary TB

Widespread haematological spread of bacilli.

## Symptoms

1 Night sweats
2 Weight loss
3 Cough
4 Haemoptysis
5 Pleural effusion
6 Meningitis.

## Diagnosis

1 CXR (upper-lobe shadowing, loss of volume, cavitation)
2 Sputum examination for acid-alcohol-fast bacilli (AAFBs)
3 Early morning urine for AAFBs
4 Lymph node biopsy
5 Bone marrow aspirate
6 Bronchoscopy and lavage
7 Culture takes at least six weeks.

## Treatment

1 In HIV-negative Caucasians with no previous treatment or contact, triple therapy with rifampicin, isoniazid and pyrazinamide
2 Others – add ethambutol
3 Triple/quadruple therapy for two months, then rifampicin and isoniazid for a further four months
4 Compliance very important
5 Side effects common:
   (a) Rifampicin:
       (i)   Hepatitis
       (ii)  Pink/orange urine
       (iii) Enzyme inducer
   (b) Isoniazid:
       (i)   Hepatitis
       (ii)  Peripheral neuropathy (cover with pyridoxine)
   (c) Pyrazinamide:
       (i)   Hepatitis
       (ii)  Rash
       (iii) Gout
   (d) Ethambutol:
       (i)   Optic neuritis

  (ii) Renal dysfunction.

Multidrug-resistant TB – 2% of all cases.

# Miscellaneous respiratory topics and lists

### Obstructive sleep apnoea

1 Incidence 1–2%, middle-aged men
2 Ten or more episodes of apnoea of at least ten seconds duration per hour
3 Occurs in REM sleep
4 Airway obstruction at base of tongue/soft palate due to loss of muscle tone
5 Symptoms of daytime somnolence, snoring and headaches
6 Causes are obesity (80%), acromegaly, hypothyroidism, alcohol
7 Diagnosis – Epworth sleep score and overnight pulse oximetry
8 Treatment is weight loss and nasal CPAP.

### Pleural effusion

1 Transudate (protein < 30 g/l):
 (a) Cardiac failure
 (b) Cirrhosis
 (c) Hypoalbuminaemia
 (d) Nephrotic syndrome
 (e) Hypothyroidism
 (f) Dialysis
2 Exudate (protein > 30 g/l):
 (a) Parapneumonic
 (b) TB
 (c) Subphrenic abscess
 (d) Pulmonary embolus
 (e) Pancreatitis (amylase in fluid)
 (f) Asbestos
 (g) Rheumatoid disease (RF in fluid)
 (h) SLE
 (i) Malignancy
3 Low fluid glucose in:
 (a) Rheumatoid arthritis

(b) TB
(c) Malignancy
(d) Empyema.

## Causes of haemoptysis

1 Lung cancer
2 TB
3 Pulmonary embolus
4 Bronchiectasis
5 Aspergilloma
6 Pulmonary abscess
7 Farmer's lung
8 Wegener's granulomatosis
9 Goodpasture's syndrome
10 Polyarteritis nodosa.

## Cavitation on CXR

1 Bullae
2 Pneumonias (*Klebsiella*, staphylococcal, anaerobic)
3 TB
4 Abscess
5 Tumour (squamous cell, secondaries)
6 Pulmonary embolus
7 Pneumoconiotic nodule
8 Rheumatoid nodule
9 Wegener's granulomatosis
10 Churg–Strauss syndrome
11 Honeycomg lung (systemic sclerosis)
12 Progressive massive fibrosis.

## Calcification on CXR

1 Lung:
  (a) TB
  (b) Carcinoma
  (c) Chickenpox
  (d) Sarcoid
  (e) Asbestos exposure
  (f) Silicosis

    (g)  Pneumoconiosis
    (h)  Hydatid disease
    (i)  Schistosomiasis
2  Pleura:
    (a)  Asbestos
    (b)  Empyema
    (c)  Haemothorax
    (d)  TB
    (e)  Recurrent pneumothorax
3  Lymph nodes:
    (a)  TB
    (b)  Carcinoid
    (c)  Silicosis
4  Other sites:
    (a)  Pericardium
    (b)  Heart valves
    (c)  Aorta.

# Rheumatology

## Common causes of an acute monoarthritis

1  Acute septic arthritis
2  Gout
3  Pseudogout
4  Trauma
5  Seronegative spondyloarthritides
6  Rheumatoid arthritis (RA)
7  Haemarthrosis.

## Causes of an acute polyarthritis

1  RA
2  Osteoarthritis (OA), generalised
3  Viral infections:
   (a)  Rubella
   (b)  Mumps
   (c)  Parvovirus
   (d)  Coxsackie
   (e)  Hepatitis B and C
4  Reiter's syndrome
5  Seronegative arthritides
6  Gonococcal arthritis
7  Adult- and childhood-onset Still's disease
8  Rheumatic fever
9  Systemic lupus erythematosus (SLE)
10  Gout (10% are polyarthropathy)
11  Pyrophosphate arthropathy
12  Acute sarcoidosis.

**Characteristics of synovial fluid in health and disease**

Table 33

| Source | Colour/ Culture | Clarity | Viscosity | WCC ($\times 10^6$/litre) |
|---|---|---|---|---|
| Normal | Yellow/ Negative | Clear | High | <200 |
| OA | Yellow/ Negative | Clear | High | <200 |
| RA | Yellow-green/ Negative | Clear/turbid | Low | 3000–50,000 |
| Bacterial arthritis | Purulent/ Positive | Turbid | Low | 50,000–100,000 |
| Gout | Yellow-white/ Negative | Clear | Low | 100–150,000 |
| Pseudogout | Yellow-white/ Negative | Clear/ bloodstained | Low | 50–75,000 |

# Bacteria associated with septic arthritis

1 *Staphylococcus aureus*
2 *Streptococcus pyogenes*
3 *Streptococcus pneumoniae*
4 *Mycobacterium tuberculosis*
5 *Neisseria gonorrhoeae*
6 *Salmonella* spp.

# Crystal-related arthropathies

## Gout

1 Arthropathy due to deposition of monosodium urate crystals in joints
2 Diagnosed by finding crystals in joints
3 Crystals are needle-shaped and negatively birefringent
4 Most commonly affects first metatarsophalangeal joint
5 Can affect any joint

6 Causes of gout:
  (a) Increased production of urate:
    (i) Increased purine synthesis:
      • Idiopathic
      • Lesch–Nyhan syndrome (X-linked)
    (ii) Increased turnover of preformed purines:
      • Lymphoproliferative and myeloproliferative disorders
      • Cytotoxic drugs
      • Chronic haemolytic anaemias
  (b) Decreased excretion of urate:
    (i) Idiopathic
    (ii) Chronic renal failure
    (iii) Increased level of organic acids (alcohol, starvation, exercise, ketoacidosis)
  (c) Drugs:
    (i) Diuretics – thiazides and furosemide (frusemide)
    (i) Salicylates (low-dose)
7 Treatment:
  (a) Acute:
    (i) NSAIDs, e.g. diclofenac
    (i) Colchicine
    (i) Steroids (systemic or intra-articular)
  (b) Prevention: allopurinol (xanthine-oxidase inhibitor).

## Pyrophosphate arthropathy (pseudogout)

1 Arthropathy due to crystals of calcium pyrophosphate
2 Crystals are positively birefringent
3 Usually causes large joint arthropathy, e.g. knees
4 X-ray will show calcium deposition in the joint (chondrocalcinosis)
5 Causes:
  (a) Older age
  (b) OA
  (c) Familial
  (d) Diabetes mellitus
  (e) Acromegaly
  (f) Haemochromatosis
  (g) Hypothyroidism
  (h) Hyperparathyroidism
6 Treatment – symptomatic.

# Rheumatoid arthritis (RA)

1 This is an autoimmune chronic inflammatory polyarthropathy
2 Revised American College of Rheumatology criteria for the classification of rheumatoid arthritis (1987) – a diagnosis of RA may be made if at least four of these seven criteria are present:
   (a) Morning stiffness (>1 hour) for > 6 weeks
   (b) Arthritis of three or more joint areas for > 6 weeks
   (c) Arthritis of the hand joints for > 6 weeks
   (d) Symmetrical arthritis
   (e) Rheumatoid nodules
   (f) Serum rheumatoid factor
   (g) Radiographic changes
3 Joint involvement in RA – symmetrical polyarthropathy affecting:
   (a) MCP joints 90%
   (b) PIP joints 90%
   (c) MTP joints 90%
   (d) Wrists 80%
   (e) Knees 80%
   (f) Ankle/subtalar 80%
   (g) Shoulder 60%
   (h) Hip 50%
   (i) Elbow 50%
   (j) Cervical spine 40%
4 Features of rheumatoid hands:
   (a) Symmetrical deforming polyarthropathy affecting MCP, PIP and wrist joints
   (b) Spares DIP joints
   (c) Active joints are hot, swollen and tender
   (d) Ulnar deviation at MCP joints
   (e) Subluxation at MCP joints and wrist
   (f) Swan-neck deformity
   (g) Boutonnière deformity
   (h) Z deformity of thumbs
   (i) Wasting of dorsal interossei
   (j) Absence of psoriatic nail changes
   (k) Nail fold infarcts or vasculitic lesions
   (l) Evidence of carpal tunnel syndrome
   (m) Palmar erythema

5 Extra-articular features of RA:
  (a) Non-organ-specific:
    (i) Weight loss
    (ii) Fever
    (iii) Lymphadenopathy
    (iv) Rheumatoid nodules (patients will be RF-positive)
    (v) Felty's syndrome
    (vi) Amyloidosis
    (vii) Increased susceptibility to infections
    (viii) Osteoporosis
  (b) Organ-specific:
    (i) Cardiac:
      • Pericarditis and effusion
      • Valvular heart disease
    (ii) Pulmonary:
      • Pleurisy
      • Pleural effusion
      • Interstitial fibrosis
      • Nodular lung disease
      • Caplan's syndrome (nodules and progressive massive fibrosis in coal workers)
    (iii) Neurological:
      • Compressive neuropathies, e.g. carpal tunnel syndrome
      • Mononeuritis multiplex (vasculitis)
      • Cervical myelopathies
    (iv) Renal:
      • Amyloidosis
      • Drug-induced glomerulonephritis or interstitial nephritis
    (v) Ocular:
      • Episcleritis and scleritis
      • Scleromalacia perforans
      • Sjögren's syndrome
6 Laboratory findings in RA:
  (a) Anaemia – normochromic or hypochromic, normocytic
  (b) Thrombocytosis
  (c) Raised ESR
  (d) Raised CRP
  (e) Raised ferritin
  (f) Low iron concentration
  (g) Low TIBC

(h)  Raised globulins
(i)   Raised ALP
(j)   Rheumatoid factor:
  • Autoantibodies against the Fc component of IgG antibodies
  • Positive in 80% of RA patients
  • Found in 5% of the general population (up to 25% in over-75s)

7  Radiological features in RA:
  (a)  Soft-tissue swelling
  (b)  Loss of joint space due to erosion of articular cartilage
  (c)  Juxta-articular osteoporosis
  (d)  Marginal bone erosions
  (e)  Joint deformities

8  Drug treatments for RA:
  (a)  Symptom-modifying drugs:
    (i)   Analgesics
    (ii)  NSAIDs
  (b)  Disease-modifying drugs:
    (i)    Antimalarials
    (ii)   Sulfasalazine
    (iii)  Gold
    (iv)   Penicillamine
    (v)    Corticosteroids
    (vi)   Methotrexate
    (vii)  Azathioprine
    (viii) Ciclosporin
    (ix)   Infliximab.

# Seronegative spondyloarthritides

Associated with HLA-B27.
1  Ankylosing spondylitis
2  Psoriatic arthritis
3  Enteropathic arthritis – Crohn's, UC, Whipples disease
4  Reiter's syndrome/reactive arthritis.

## Comparison of seronegative spondyloarthritides and seropositive RA

**Table 34**

|  | Seronegative | Seropositive |
|---|---|---|
| Peripheral arthritis | Asymmetrical | Symmetrical |
| Spinal involvement | Ankylosis | Cervical subluxation |
| Cartilaginous joints | Commonly affected (SI joints) | Rarely affected |
| Tissue typing | HLA-B27 | (HLA-DR4) |
| Eye | Anterior uveitis Conjunctivitis | Scleritis |
| Skin | Psoriasis Keratoderma blenorrhagica Mucosal ulceration Erythema nodosum | Cutaneous nodules Vasculitis |
| Heart | Aortic regurgitation Conduction defects | Pericarditis |
| Pulmonary | Chest wall ankylosis Apical fibrosis | Nodules Effusions Fibrosis |
| Gastrointestinal | Ulceration of small or large intestine | Drug-induced symptoms |
| Genitourinary | Urethritis Genital ulceration |  |

## Common features of seronegative spondyloarthritides

1 Negative RF
2 Asymmetrical inflammatory peripheral arthritis (oligoarthritis)
3 Radiological sacroiliitis
4 Spondylitis
5 Enthesitis
6 HLA-B27 association (96% in ankylosing spondylitis)
7 Anterior uveitis
8 Evidence of clinical overlap between diseases.

## Ankylosing spondylitis

### Clinical features (the 'A' disease)

1 **A**rthritis
2 **A**nterior uveitis
3 **A**pical pulmonary fibrosis
4 **A**myloidosis
5 **A**ortic regurgitation
6 **A**ortitis.

### Radiological features

1 Sacroiliac joints:
   (a) Irregular joint margins
   (b) Sclerosis and fusion
2 Spine:
   (a) Loss of lumbar lordosis
   (b) Vertebral squaring
   (c) Syndesmophyte formation (calcification of the annulus fibrosis)
   (d) Bamboo spine (calcification in anterior and posterior spinal ligaments)
3 Peripheral joints: erosive arthropathy.

## Reiter's syndrome/reactive arthritis

### Triggers

1 *Chlamydia trachomatis*
2 *Campylobacter jejuni*
3 *Salmonella* spp.
4 *Shigella flexneri*
5 *Neisseria gonorrhoeae*
6 *Borrelia burgdorferi*.

### Clinical features

HLA-B27 80%.
1 Classical triad:
   (a) Arthropathy
   (b) Conjunctivitis
   (c) Urethritis

2 Other features:
   (a) Sacroiliitis
   (b) Plantar fasciitis
   (c) Circinate balanitis
   (d) Keratoderma blenorrhagica
   (e) Oral ulceration
   (f) Pericarditis.

## Psoriatic arthropathy

1 Peripheral oligoarthritis or polyarthritis (60%)
2 Spondylitis (15%)
3 Distal interphalangeal disease (10%)
4 Rheumatoid type (10%)
5 Arthritis mutilans (5%).

## Treatment for spondyloarthropathies

1 Physiotherapy
2 Local steroid injection
3 NSAIDs
4 Systemic steroids
5 Sulfasalazine
6 Methotrexate
7 Antibiotics (acute infections).

# Connective tissue diseases

## Systemic lupus erythematosus (SLE)

### Diagnosis

The American College of Rheumatology revised criteria for the diagnosis of SLE (1982) state that SLE may be diagnosed in the presence of four or more of the following:
   1 Malar rash
   2 Discoid rash
   3 Photosensitivity
   4 Oral ulcers
   5 Arthritis

6  Serositis (pleurisy, pericarditis)
7  Renal disease (persistent proteinuria > 0.5g/day, cellular casts)
8  Neurological disorder (seizures, psychosis)
9  Haematological disorder (haemolytic anaemia, leucopenia, lymphopenia, thrombocytopenia)
10 Immunological disorder (LE cells, Anti-dsDNA antibody, anti-Sm anitbody or false-positive VDRL)
11 Antinuclear antibody.

## Clinical features

1  Mucocutaneous (81%):
   (a)  Rash (malar, discoid, photosensitive)
   (b)  Alopecia
   (c)  Oral, nasal, or vaginal ulcers
   (d)  Raynaud's phenomenon (50%)
   (e)  Livedo reticularis
   (f)  Cutaneous vasculitis
   (g)  Sjögren's syndrome
2  Musculoskeletal (95%):
   (a)  Migratory asymmetrical non-erosive (Jaccoud's) arthritis
   (b)  Myalgia and myositis
3  Renal (53%):
   (a)  Glomerulonephritis
   (b)  Nephrotic syndrome
   (c)  Hypertension
   (d)  End-stage renal failure (<5%)
4  Respiratory (48%):
   (a)  Pleurisy
   (b)  Recurrent pneumontis
   (c)  Pulmonary hypertension
5  Cardiovascular (38%):
   (a)  Pericarditis
   (b)  Cardiomyopathy
   (c)  Myocarditis
   (d)  Libman–Sacks endocarditis
6  Neurological disease (59%):
   (a)  Migraine
   (b)  Seizures
   (c)  Chorea

(d) Psychosis
(e) CVA (vasculitis)
(f) Mononeuritis multiplex
7 Haematological:
  (a) Neutropenia
  (b) Lymphopenia
  (c) Thrombocytopenia
  (d) Lymphadenopathy
  (e) Splenomegaly
  (f) Antiphospholipid syndrome
8 Gastrointestinal:
  (a) Mesenteric vasculitis
  (b) Chronic active hepatitis.

### Typical investigation results

1 Normochromic normocytic anaemia with active disease
2 Leucopenia/lymphopenia
3 Raised ESR
4 Normal CRP (unless accompanied by serositis, synovitis or infection)
5 ANA positive in 95%
6 Raised immunoglobulins
7 Low C3 and C4
8 Antiphospholipid antibodies in 30–40%
9 Coombs-positive haemolytic anaemia.

### Causes of a positive ANA

1 SLE (95%)
2 Sjögren's syndrome (80%)
3 Polymyositis/dermatomyositis (80%)
4 RA (30%)
5 Autoimmune hepatitis.

### Treatment

1 Sunscreens – photosensitivity
2 NSAIDs – symptomatic
3 Chloroquine/hydroxychloroquine – rashes, arthritis, malaise
4 Corticosteroids – severe flare, low-dose for maintenance
5 Immunosuppressives (azathioprine, methotrexate,

cyclophosphamide) – for severe flare

6  Plasma exchange – severe cases
7  Anticoagulation – recurrent thromboses
8  Vasodilators (calcium blockers, prostacyclin) – Raynaud's
9  Antihypertensives.

## Antiphospholipid antibody syndrome

1  IgG or IgM antibodies against phospholipids
2  Antibodies may cause a false-positive VDRL
3  *In vitro* anticoagulant effect – prolonged APTT which fails to correct after addition of normal plasma
4  Predisposes to recurrent thromboses *in vivo*
5  Clinical features:
    (a)  Venous thrombosis – DVT
    (b)  Arterial thrombosis – MI, CVA, etc.
    (c)  Other features:
        (i)   Recurrent miscarriage
        (ii)  Thrombocytopenia
        (iii) Livedo reticularis
        (iv)  Pulmomary hypertension.

## Systemic sclerosis (scleroderma)

### Diffuse systemic sclerosis

1  Truncal and forearm skin involvement
2  Anti-Scl-70 antibodies in 30%.

### Limited systemic sclerosis

1  Skin involvement limited to hands, face, feet and forearms, or absent
2  Includes CREST syndrome (**c**alcinosis, **R**aynaud's, o**e**sophageal involvement, **s**clerodactyly and **t**elangiectasia)
3  High incidence of anticentromere antibody (70–80%).

### Clinical features

1  Musculoskeletal:
    (a)  Polyarthralgia
    (b)  Polymyositis
2  Skin:

   (a)  Raynaud's phenomenon (almost all patients)
   (b)  Abnormal nail-fold capillaries
   (c)  Sclerodactyly
   (d)  Telangiectasia
   (e)  Tight smooth waxy pigmented skin
   (f)  Skin ulcers
   (g)  Subcutaneous calcification
3 Heart:
   (a)  Cardiomyopathy
   (b)  Pericarditis
   (c)  Hypertension
4 Pulmonary:
   (a)  Pulmonary fibrosis
   (b)  Pulmonary hypertension
5 Gastrointestinal:
   (a)  Microstomia
   (b)  Dysphagia – poor motility, peptic strictures
   (c)  GORD – low sphincter pressure, hiatus hernia
   (d)  Diverticulae – small bowel, colonic
   (e)  Bacterial overgrowth and malabsorption
6 Renal:
   (a)  Progressive renal failure
   (b)  Hypertensive renal crisis.

## Raynaud's phenomenon

1 Episodic event characterised by the digits turning white and numb, then cyanosed, and finally red and painful (rebound hyperaemia)
2 3–10% of adults affected
3 1% of Raynaud's sufferers have a connective tissue disorder
4 Causes:
   (a)  Idiopathic
   (b)  Connective tissue disorders
   (c)  Cervical rib
   (d)  Increased plasma viscosity
   (e)  Drugs (beta blockers)
   (f)  Vibrating instruments
5 Treatment:
   (a)  Warmth
   (b)  No smoking or beta-blockers

(c)  Calcium-channel blockers
(d)  GTN
(e)  Prostacyclin infusion.

**Autoantibodies in connective tissue diseases**

**Table 35**

| Antibody | Disease |
| --- | --- |
| Anti-dsDNA | SLE |
| Anti-Sm | SLE |
| Anti-Ro | Sjögren's, SLE |
| Anti-La | Sjögren's, SLE |
| Anti-RNP | Mixed connective tissue disease, SLE |
| Anti-Jo-1 | Polymyositis |
| Anti-Scl-70 | Diffuse cutaneous systemic sclerosis |
| Anticentromere | Limited cutaneous systemic sclerosis |
| Anticardiolipin | Antiphospholipid antibody syndrome, SLE |
| Antihistones | Drug-induced lupus |

# Juvenile chronic arthritis

1  Arthritis in at least one joint for over three months
2  Onset before 16 years
3  Exclusion of other diseases that may cause arthritis
4  Still's disease (10%) is the systemic form:
   (a)  Fever
   (b)  Evanescent, macular, erythematous rash (salmon-pink)
   (c)  Arthritis (usually the systemic features precede arthritis).

# Revised Jones Criteria for diagnosis of acute rheumatic fever

## Major criteria

1  Carditis
2  Polyarthritis
3  Chorea

4 Erythema marginatum
5 Subcutaneous nodules.

**Minor criteria**

1 Fever
2 Arthralgia
3 Previous history of rheumatic fever or rheumatic heart disease.

Diagnosis requires two major, or one major and two minor, plus evidence of recent streptococcal infection (raised ASO titre or culture of group A streptorocci).

# Risk factors for osteoarthritis

1 Age
2 Female sex
3 Genetic predisposition
4 Obesity
5 Hypermobility
6 Joint trauma – particularly fractures through the joint
7 Chondrocalcinosis
8 Septic arthritis
9 Developmental conditions:
    (a) Congenital dislocation of the hip
    (b) Perthes disease
10 Bone disease – Paget's disease
11 Endocrine conditions:
    (a) Acromegaly
    (b) Haemochromatosis
    (c) Wilson's disease.

# Vasculitis

## Large vessel

1 Takayasu's arteritis:
    (a) Often presents with arm claudication and pulseless vessels
    (b) Diagnosis by angiography

2  Giant cell arteritis:
  (a)  Typically involves extracranial arteries, leading to ischaemia
  (b)  Important treatable cause of loss of vision in the elderly
  (c)  Raised ESR
  (d)  Diagnosis by temporal artery biopsy (a negative biopsy does not exclude diagnosis, however)
  (e)  Easily treated with steroids
  (f)  Clinical features:
      (i)   Unilateral throbbing headache
      (ii)  Jaw claudication
      (iii) Amaurosis fugax
      (iv)  Diplopia
      (v)   Polymyalgia rheumatica symptoms in 50%.

## Medium vessel

1  Polyarteritis nodosa (PAN):
  (a)  Associated with hepatitis B infection
  (b)  American College of Rheumatology criteria for diagnosis of PAN:
      (i)    Weight loss of over 4 kg
      (ii)   Livedo reticularis
      (iii)  Testicular pain
      (iv)   Myalgia/leg tenderness
      (v)    Mono/polyneuropathy
      (vi)   Hepatitis Bs Ag positive
      (vii)  Arteriographic abnormality
      (viii) Positive biopsy
2  Kawasaki disease:
  (a)  Vasculitis primarily in children under five years
  (b)  Coronary artery lesions (aneurysms) in 40% can lead to sudden death, MI or papillary muscle dysfunction
  (c)  Treatment is with aspirin and high-dose gammaglobulin (reduces mortality from 30% to less than 1%).

## Small vessel

1  Churg–Strauss syndrome:
  (a)  Asthma
  (b)  Eosinophilia
  (c)  Systemic vasculitis

2 Wegener's granulomatosis:
   (a) cANCA positive in over 95%
   (b) Characterised by upper respiratory tract lesions, pulmonary disease and glomerulonephritis
3 Microscopic polyangiitis:
   (a) Vasculitis affecting single organ or multisystems
   (b) pANCA positive
4 Henoch–Schönlein purpura:
   (a) Most common systemic vasculitis in children
   (b) IgA deposited in skin and kidney
   (c) Preceded by upper respiratory tract infection in 90%
   (d) Clinical features:
      (i) Purpuric rash (100%) – lower limbs and buttocks
      (ii) Arthralgia
      (iii) Glomerulonephritis
      (iv) Gastrointestinal bleeding
      (v) Intussusception.

## Treatment of vasculitis

1 Aggressive immunosuppression:
   (a) Initially – pulsed methylprednisolone and cyclophosphamide, plus high-dose steroids
   (b) Maintenance – steroids, azathioprine
2 Plasma exchange may be necessary.

## Polymyalgia rheumatica

1 Most common in patients aged 60–70 years
2 25% have giant cell arteritis
3 Raised ESR and ALP (30%)
4 Symptoms and ESR respond rapidly to steroids
5 Clinical features (often sudden onset):
   (a) Proximal muscle weakness, worse in the morning
   (b) Weight loss
   (c) Joint pain
   (d) Symptoms of giant cell arteritis (see above).

## Malignant tumours of bone

[see Table 36, opposite]

## Causes of a very high ESR (> 100 mm/hour)

1 Multiple myeloma
2 Giant cell arteritis/polymyalgia rheumatical
3 Sepsis
4 Occult malignancy
5 SLE.

### Side effects of anti-rheumatoid drugs

1 Hydroxychloroquine:
  (a) Pigmentation
  (b) Maculopathy
  (c) Leucopenia
2 Gold:
  (a) Dermatitis (30%)
  (b) Proteinuria and glomerulonephritis
  (c) Thrombocytopenia
  (d) Leucopenia
  (e) Aplastic anaemia
3 Penicillamine:
  (a) Maculopapular rash
  (b) Loss of taste sensation
  (c) Proteinura and nephrotic syndrome
  (d) Drug-induced lupus
  (e) Myasthenia gravis
  (f) Thrombocytopenia
  (g) Pancytopenia
4 Sulfazalazine
  (a) Nausea
  (b) Skin rashes
  (c) Hepatitis
  (d) Pulmonary eosinophilia

**Table 36**

| Tumour | Age | Common sites | Behaviour | Treatment and prognosis |
| --- | --- | --- | --- | --- |
| Osteosarcoma | Young adults | Long bones, esp. distal femur and proximal tibia | Rapid growth, pain and swelling, lung metastases | Surgery and chemotherapy 40% cure rate |
| Chondrosarcoma | 35–60 years | Pelvis, ribs, spine, long bones | Slow enlargement, eventual vascular invasion | Surgery 75% cure rate |
| Fibrosarcoma and malignant fibrous histiocytoma | Any age, peak 30–40 years | Femur, tibia, humerus, pelvis | Local growth, vascular invasion | Surgery 40% cure rate |
| Ewing's sarcoma | Children and teenagers | Long bones, pelvis and ribs | Widespread metastases | Chemotherapy 10% cure rate |

  (e) Macrocytosis
  (f) Haemolytic anaemia
  (g) Pancytopenia
  (h) Reduced sperm (reversible)
5 Methotrexate:
  (a) Hepatic fibrosis
  (b) Blood dyscrasias
6 Cyclophosphamide:
  (a) Haemorrhagic cystitis
  (b) Pancytopenia.

# Index